Autophagy Fasting With Water for Beginners

How to Master the Art of Weight Loss and Discover the Amazing Diet Secrets Behind the Power of Fasting! Lose Weight, Live Healthy, and Feel Younger!

Jason Berg

Eric Fung

Table of Contents

Introduction

Autophagy ranks high among the most popular methods of weight management and healthy living, and this process is termed autophagy for a reason. Most people who have tried it can relate the benefits they have derived and the ways it has improved their life. But then, what is autophagy?

Do you suffer from recurrent body pains? Are you easily prone to illness, or do you find it difficult to shed some weight? Then, all you need to do is to acquire more knowledge of autophagy and the fasting processed involved.

This book will enlighten you on what autophagy is all about, the benefits associated with it and many more.

- Here is a clue of what lies ahead:
- All about autophagy; how it works, how to induce it, and its benefits
- Benefits and side effects of fasting, and precautions to take when fasting
- Myths about Water Fasting and Autophagy
- Water Fasting; its types, benefits, and how to harness it for all its benefits
- How to ease into fasting, doing it the right and easy way, and understanding your routine

Everyone needs autophagy in their lives, and no one benefits from being overweight; rather, being overweight poses some health risks. Being overweight can cause inflammation, heart-related diseases as well as others.

Can you imagine how active and alive you will feel after losing some weight within a few weeks into autophagy? Furthermore, imagine how happy your friends and family will be when they see you radiating with more energy than ever before? All these benefits can be achieved with less stress and without starving yourself to death.

Autophagy and water fasting are the best choices for those who wish to have a healthy and clean body.

Chapter 1: Autophagy/Water Fasting

Over time, the metabolic activities in a healthy human body lead to cellular damage. Sadly, the rate at which our cells are damaged increases as we age due to stress, exposure to radiation among others. However, Autophagy can help the body remove such damaged cells as well as old cells that are no longer active but are still present in the body. If such cells are not removed, it may lead to inflammatory diseases as well as other harmful cardiovascular diseases.

Autophagy is derived from the combination of two Greek words which are: **auto** which means 'self' and **phagy** which means to 'engulf.' Therefore, autophagy means the engulfment of the body's cells or tissues as part of the normal metabolic processes which is both beneficial and protective.

Over the years, fasting has been used as a way of shedding weight.

The fast diet also known as water fasting or water cleanse, involves the consumption of water alone over a specific period, with no calories intake at all for a set period. This fast is in stark contrast with caloric restriction in which the daily consumption is cut down to about 20 to 40%.

What you eat during a water fast?

When doing a water fast, you can't by any means eat anything. Also, you are not expected to drink something else besides water. In water fasting, the average daily intake of water is about 2-3 liters.

This fast should last for at least 24 hours, and 72 hours at most. Water fasting beyond this period requires guidance and supervision by medical professionals because some health risks might come with it. It is typical of water fast to make you feel weak and dizzy. However, try not to get involved in any overwhelming physical work. Also, stay away from long-distance driving to avoid an accident.

NB:

- *In water fasting, everything is forbidden except water, and it usually lasts for 24-72 hours.*

- *Do not exceed this period without proper medical monitoring.*

In recent times, this method of fasting has become more popular as an effective way of shedding weight.

Some of the reasons why people go on a water fast:

- For religious purpose
- For weight loss
- For detoxification
- For its associated health benefits
- For those preparing for a medical treatment

However, most people go on water fasting primarily because of its associated health benefits.

The Origin of Autophagy

Early in the 1950s, Christian de Duve a Belgian scientist discovered the process of autophagy by accident while working on insulin.

Between 1970 and 1980, researchers began taking a closer look at the process of cellular autophagy. At that time, little information was available about the importance of autophagy. After so many years of hard work, a significant milestone was achieved in 1983, when Yoshinori Ohsumi, discovered genes responsible for the regulation of autophagy in yeast. From his discovery, he found out that autophagy was absent in yeast cells lacking those genes and such cells were unable to repair themselves. In 2016, he was awarded a Nobel Prize for this great discovery.[1] [2]

The interesting thing about this discovery is how the cell responds to increased stress, nutrient deficiency, deprivation of energy and cellular injuries by increasing the rate of cellular autophagy but where the stress is eliminated, the process of autophagy goes back to the regular rate (maintenance mode).

With more desires to fully understand the process of autophagy, more research works are now aimed at understanding the relationship between aging and autophagy, and the

[1] Ohsumi, Y. (2013). Historical landmarks of autophagy research. *Cell Research*, *24*(1), 9-23. doi: 10.1038/cr.2013.169
[2] Autophagy 101: How Intermittent Fasting Could Help Us Age Slowly. (2019). Retrieved from https://thechalkboardmag.com/what-is-autophagy-intermittent-fasting-process

effect of stress on this process.

There is a general theory that there is a relationship between aging and the rate of autophagy as well. According to evidence, the process that enhances autophagy will also help to extend the lifespan of such individual. Another research reported that cell related aging attributed to the accumulation of damaged cells without proper means of removal. Since autophagy helps to remove damaged cells thereby slowing down the process of aging, scientists are looking at ways of extending the life expectancy of humans by inducing autophagy.

Benefits of Fasting:

1. **It enhances the body's fitness.** Fasting helps the body to burn fats, and as such, the body will feel lighter and such individual can be said to be fit.

2. **Promotes greater satiety.** Your adipocytes produce various hormones (acting as an endocrine organ), such as your leptin which regulates the way you feel. When you fast; however, you burn most of these stored fatty tissues, your leptin levels drop automatically (creating a leptin-deficient environment). Hence, whenever the little amount of leptin is produced, the effect is heightened, and your body becomes more responsive to leptin thereby modulating how you feel after a meal.

3. **Enhanced metabolism.** Leptin is also known as the (satiety hormone) also stimulate the production of thyroid hormones. Thus, enhanced leptin responsiveness will directly increase the rate of metabolism.

4. **Facilitates fat loss and ketosis.** Fat-loss or ketosis can be accomplished either by eating a Ketogenic Diet or by fasting. A Ketogenic Diet helps to burn out stored fat which is harmful rather than helpful to the body organs such as the liver, the kidneys, and the blood vessels.

5. **Enhances insulin sensitivity:** When you fast, the body secretes a lesser amount of insulin which in turn increases insulin sensitivity.

6. **Boosts cardiovascular health:** Fasting is recommended for those who wish to improve their cardiovascular function and have normal blood pressure.

7. **Reduced blood pressure.** Most people experience lower BP while fasting. This effect could be as a result of lower salt consumption and increased salt loss through urine.

8. **Lower blood sugar.** The blood sugar could drop as much as over 30 percent within a few days of fasting, and if care is not taken, the person could become hyperglycemic.

9. **Decreases blood triglycerides.** The triglycerides content of the blood drops low while an individual is fasting which helps to increase the blood flow within the blood vessels which could have been narrowed by fat components.

10. **Better heart condition.** Fasting has been found to help reduce the accumulation of free radicals within the body. Free radicals are harmful to the muscles of the heart.

11. **Could slow the rate of aging and prolong your lifespan.** There have been positive results obtained from animal studies to prove that fasting could prolong lifespan. Also, when the blood is cleaned regularly, it slows down the process of aging and improves the health of an individual.

12. **Suppresses inflammation.** Although several factors cause inflammation, an unhealthy diet could lead to increased production of free radicals which in turn could cause inflammation. Food items such as alcohol, refined food items, fried foods, etc. are all sources of free radicals.

13. **Reduces the effects of Oxidative Stress.** When the rate at which free radicals are produced is higher than the rate at which it is eliminated, it accumulates in the body thereby causing oxidative stress which is damaging to the cells of the body.

14. **Enhances cellular recycling process.** Senescent cells accumulate in our body as we age. But when we fast, the body activates the process of self-digestion, and along the line, malignant cells are also destroyed.

15. **Growth regulation.** It has been found that insulin-like growth factor 1 (IGF-1) could lead to the proliferation of cancer. But fasting suppresses the production of IGF-1.

16. **Protects the brain.** Research works carried out on the function of the brain and aging have revealed one could age gracefully by fasting regularly.

17. **Promotes a healthy stress response.** Moderate stress is beneficial to the brain especially when it is infrequent, and fasting can induce such stress. Moderate stress triggers a series of activities that are protective to the brain cells (neurons).

18. **Promotes recovery from an injury.** Though the mechanism is not fully understood, research from animal models has shown that intermittent fasting

helps the healing process.

19. **Supports healthier skin collagen production.** Your skin is a reflection of your diet. Accumulation of glucose can compromise the structure of the collagen, but fasting can help you overcome this challenge and give your skin that glow.

Side Effects of Fasting

Everyone fasts for various reasons such as: to lose weight, for a religious purpose, for healthy living and the list goes on. A fast could either be mild or strict (ranging from liquid only such as juice, tea, coffee and the likes to no food, no fluid). Although fasting comes with a lot of benefits, it also has its associated downsides which could either be short term or long term. These effects vary from one individual to another.

Poor weight management. Many people tend to crave for and consume more calories after a long period of fasting which will inevitably counteract all the progress made by fasting.

Short-term downsides. Fasting could have several adverse effects such: dizziness, headaches, outbursts, weakness, low blood pressure, gouts/gall stones among others.

Long-Term downsides. Continuous prolonged fasting could weaken the immune system and affect vital organs such as the kidneys and the liver. When an individual abstains from food over a long period, he becomes malnourished and could lead to an untimely death after the entire energy store of the body has been exhausted.

Dry Fast. Dry fasting is the most dangerous form of fasting in which an individual abstains from food and fluids. It could even lead to death if other underlying factors such as exertions, heat and the likes set in.

Water Fasting. There is a high tendency of losing the wrong type of weight while performing this form of fasting. This is because this form of fasting only allows the intake of water but restrict one from taking in calories. Although an individual could lose up to 0.9kg (2 pounds) 24-72 hours of water fasting, sadly, such weight loss can be a loss of carbohydrates, muscle mass and even water.

Possible dehydration. As funny as it may sound, water fasting could still cause dehydration because about 20-30 percent of our daily water intake comes from the food we eat. Thus, if we consume the same amount of water as we do on average days, we could experience some symptoms of dehydration such as light-headedness, dizziness, constipation, headaches, weakness, nausea, etc. To prevent such unwanted side effects, you may need to increase your water consumption.

Possibility of experiencing Orthostatic Hypotension. This type of hypotension is usually common among those whose fast. You might have experienced something similar when you get up suddenly, and then you feel dizzy or lightheaded. That feeling is caused by a sudden drop in the blood pressure, and such ones are prone to fainting. If you think you are experiencing orthostatic hypotension, then it means your body is not compatible with water fasting.

Water fasting could worsen a medical condition: Those with certain medical conditions should avoid water fasting as it could worsen such conditions:

- **Gout**: Gout is caused by an accumulation of Uric acid in the joints, and water fasting could increase its production.

- **Diabetes**: In Type I and type II diabetes, fasting could aggravate the side effect of diabetes.

- **Chronic kidney disease**: Those with chronic kidney condition should avoid water fast as it may worsen such condition.

- **Eating disorders**: Bulimia nervosa could be enhanced by fasting. There is more than sufficient evidence to back this up.

- **Heartburn:** Heartburn may be induced by fasting as the body will keep producing gastric acid which helps the digestion process.

Precautions to Take When Fasting

Fasting has a lot of advantages. However, fasting is not meant for everyone. To better understand the theory of fasting, let us compare Fasting to a tool (such as an arrow) which can either be used properly or misused. Holding to that, we will use the archery metaphor to explain the effective use and the misuse of fasting/autophagy. A hunter could have different sizes and tips of arrows in his quiver. When he finds an antelope, he will use a sharp wooden arrow, but when faced by a lion or bear, he would go for something stronger: probably an arrow with metallic tips. The point is don't use the wrong method for the right purpose.

Who should avoid fasting

Pregnant and breastfeeding mothers. Whether you have a child you're breastfeeding or one who is still in your uterus, you need all the calories you can get; both the mother and the infant need to be fed well to stay nourished and healthy.

Underaged students and those below 18 should avoid Fasting. Children under the age of 18 are still growing and need all the vital nutrients and minerals to have healthy growth and development.

Those that are underweight and/or malnourished. If you find it difficult to tell whether you are malnourished or not, you could ask your physician or a trusted friend. Those having an eating disorder such as bulimia are included in this category.

Individuals who have Type-2 Diabetes. Fasting has been used over the years as a means of reversing the effect of Type-2 diabetes. However, you still need to consult your physician before beginning a fast.

Who needs to be cautious?

Another group of individuals who also need to be cautious is those with occasional gastroesophageal reflux disease (GERD). Those who fall into this category need to check with their physician as well if they wish to fast and must be closely monitored.

There are solid pieces of evidence to prove that GERD could be aggravated by fasting and the symptoms could become worsened. This possible worsening is because during fasting, the stomach will be devoid of food and there will be nothing which the gastric juice would digest.

Individuals on medications need to be cautious while fasting as the fasting periods could overlap when such drugs would be taken especially those medications that would require you to eat before using them.

In addition, those on cancer therapy and other medical treatment must be cautious and should have an in-depth discussion with their physician before fasting.

Chapter 2: How Does Autophagy Work?

Forms of Autophagy

First, let us identify the three types of autophagy.[3] They are:

- **macroautophagy**
- **microautophagy**
- **chaperone-mediated autophagy**

All the three forms of autophagy involve the process of breaking down and reproducing certain specific components found within the lysosome.

Macro-autophagy: During this process, all waste materials within a cell are transported via a double membrane-bound vesicle, (an autophagosome).[4] The waste can then fuse with the cytoplasmic lysosome (forming an autolysosome).

Micro-autophagy: This is in sharp contrast with the process of macro-autophagy. In this case, the cellular wastes to be digested are not transported via a membrane, but rather, they are mopped up by the cytoplasmic lysosome itself (via the membrane). And through this process, the cell cleans itself.[5]

NB: During the process of both macro-autophagy & microautophagy, both selective and non-selective processes can be employed when the cell wants to transport large molecules to be recycled or cleaned up.

Chaperone-mediated autophagy: During this process, the cell utilizes chaperone proteins (such as Hsc-70) which are found on the surface of the lysosomal membrane. These chaperones can then bind to the desired protein thereby facilitating their movement across the selectively permeable membrane.[6]

[3] Mizushima, N., Yoshimori, T., & Ohsumi, Y. (2011). The Role of Atg Proteins in Autophagosome Formation. *Annual Review Of Cell And Developmental Biology*, 27(1), 107-132. doi: 10.1146/annurev-cellbio-092910-154005

[4] Mizushima, N., Ohsumi, Y., & Yoshimori, T. (2002). Autophagosome Formation in Mammalian Cells. Cell Structure And Function, 27(6), 421-429. doi: 10.1247/csf.27.421

[5] Castro-Obregon, S. (2019). Lysosomes, Autophagy | Learn Science at Scitable. Retrieved from https://www.nature.com/scitable/topicpage/the-discovery-of-lysosomes-and-autophagy-14199828

[6] Bandyopadhyay, U., Kaushik, S., Varticovski, L., & Cuervo, A. (2008). The Chaperone-Mediated

From a molecular point of view, the entire process of autophagy could be divided into five stages which are:

- Initiation

- Elongation

- Autophagosome formation

- Fusion

- Autolysosome formation

- Degradation

In summary, cellular components to be degraded are collected together to form a macro/large molecule which is then broken down into smaller/micro molecules such as fatty acids, amino acids, glucose, and nucleotides.

Thus, such micro molecules will be available for use by the cell to form larger molecules. This process helps to renew the cells and therefore produce healthy cells.

Cell death occurs to ensure a balance between good and healthy cells and those that are senescent.

Autophagy is a survival mechanism that is imperative to the survival of cells especially when subjected to stressful conditions such as nutrient deprivation. Also, it helps the cell eliminate toxic materials, like pathogens, infections, and damaged organelles.

Autophagy Vs. Apoptosis

Apoptosis is defined as the programmed death of a cell which occurs as part of the cell's normal activities.

But one may wonder how apoptosis is related to autophagy. Scientists believe that autophagy is a highly selective process by which a particular organelle(s) are eliminated from a cell. Also, there is tangible evidence to prove that one process does not control the other. However, there are reasons to believe that autophagy as a whole is a process of cell death that is independent of apoptosis.

Autophagy Receptor Organizes in Dynamic Protein Complexes at the Lysosomal Membrane. *Molecular And Cellular Biology*, 28(18), 5747-5763. doi: 10.1128/mcb.02070-07

Researchers are particularly interested in the association between autophagy and apoptosis because they believe that such knowledge could aid the treatment of cancer and management of neurodegenerative diseases such as Alzheimer's disease based on the capacity of both processes to regulate cell death. When such knowledge is available, autophagy could then be used as a therapeutic tool to eliminate harmful cells while protecting the healthy ones[7]

How to Induce Autophagy

Fossil evidence from the past showed strong and healthy bones and teeth of humans at an early age of our history, yet there are also evidences to show that most humans from ancient history went for days without food.

Some reasons responsible for this include:

- **They had to work to eat:** The early men had to farm or hunt before they could eat unlike today when you can easily stroll to a grocery store to buy foodstuffs.

- **They felt weak regularly:** Lack of energy is one of the primary triggers of autophagy

Here is a simple comparison between the ancient food environment and the modern food environment:

- **Most people have access to food:** Today, there is more than enough food for everyone to eat. Food is affordable and easily accessible to all.

- **People no longer have to work hard to eat:** Most of us drive down to the grocery or talk a short stroll down to the store with money in our pocket and VOOM, we can purchase high caloric food with a little amount of money. As a matter of fact, high caloric food items are the cheapest items on the shelf. We no longer have to farm or hunt before eating.

- **We can eat anytime we want:** If one is not cautious, you might find yourself munching one thing or another for most of the day.

In our modern-day society, an average individual can't go a day without taking in food substances that are capable of inducing autophagy. However, we do not engage in sufficient rigorous activities that could help expend energy to be energy deficient. In

[7] Gump, J., & Thorburn, A. (2011). Autophagy and apoptosis: what is the connection?. *Trends In Cell Biology*, 21(7), 387-392. doi: 10.1016/j.tcb.2011.03.007

simple terms, our input is not equivalent to our output (i.e., what we take in does not equate what goes out). This is in sharp contrast with the eating environment in which our ancestors lived, and if they were given similar opportunity today, they would fall over each other to have a fill. In our modern society, the most important thing we need to focus on is finding ways to activate the process of autophagy.

Autophagy occurs in virtually all the cells in our body. However, this activity is further enhanced in response to stressful activities such as hunger, and starvation. Additional activities that could be considered as adequate stressors include exercise, fasting. Research has shown that both activities have helped to prevent age-related diseases, induce weight loss, and can extend the life-span of an individual.

Four ways of inducing autophagy while carrying out your normal daily activities:

1. Fasting. Due to our hectic lifestyles, it is good to know that you can still control your eating habits and your lifestyle. One of the good triggers of autophagy isn't very hard to imagine at all. One of the more popular triggers you can practice is intermittent fasting (IMF), and you can still take other liquids such as water and tea/coffee.

What is intermittent fasting? This is a form of time-restricted fasting in which an individual abstains from food for a specified period. We have different types of intermittent fasting such as the eating window and alternate-day fasting.

How long before autophagy is triggered? Well, studies have shown that fasting for 1-2 days (24-48 hours) usually produces the best effect.[8] However, this is an impossible task for most people. Still, many people can still fast for half a day (12 hours) or more without too much trouble, and this can be done by eating once or twice daily. For instance, if you had your last meal by 7 PM today, the next meal should come by 7 AM or thereabout. That way, you would have fasted for 12 hours. You could then have the next meal by 7 PM.

Another option is to have your regular meal at regular intervals then you go on a two to three day (2–3 days) fast. When it comes to alternate fasting, you could decide to cut down on your calorie intake during the fasting periods by eating only 1–2 meals (≤500 calories) then you can have your fill of calories on regular days.

---

[8] Alirezaei, M., Kemball, C., Flynn, C., Wood, M., Whitton, J., & Kiosses, W. (2010). Short-term fasting induces profound neuronal autophagy. *Autophagy, 6*(6), 702-710. doi: 10.4161/auto.6.6.12376

Autophagy Fasting

Our bodies see any form of fasting as stress, and this sounds logical when you give it a bit of thought. During a fasting period, you feel hungry, and your body will attempt to maximize the distribution of your energy.

Below are the different kinds of fasts you can pick.

- **Long Fasts.** These type of fasts require you to stay away from any form of eating for a minimum of 24 hours.

- **Dry Fast.** This is a brutal form of fasting which remains popular despite its harshness. It is a hazardous form of fasting where you can't eat or drink anything. It is not advisable to stay away from drinking water; therefore, I would advise you to stay away from this type of fast for your health's sake.

- **Water Fast.** Water Fasting is another popular fasting type (and the reason for this book). This form of fasting is known for its autophagous, weight loss, detox, and anti-aging benefits. It requires you to stay away from eating but recommends you drink water or other forms of liquid depending on the variation of water fasting you are attempting. However, drinks such as protein shakes or juice are a "No" for it because they contain calories that could lead you to retain your weight.

Long fasts can enhance autophagy and weight loss. The loss of function by a stem cell can be reversed by one 24-hour fast, significantly improving their regeneration abilities.

You are probably thinking how long it will take you to fast to induce autophagy. Different research has shown that a fasting period of 24 to 36 hours would induce autophagy, suggesting that intermittent water fasting is another good option, although not as reliable as long water fasts, although

Fasting is about staying away from calories, to enable your body to reset its metabolic activities. This, however, doesn't mean you stay away from drinking water or specific teas, provided you don't add sugars, or you're selective about the natural sweeteners you add.

2. Ketogenic diets. Ketogenic diets (KD) are food substances that are very rich in fat but low in carbohydrates. Taking KD produces similar effects as fasting. KD comprises more than 75% of your daily fat consumption and less than 5-10% of calories obtained your daily carb consumption. When this is consumed, it triggers the body to undergo the process of gluconeogenesis (a process in which the body derives energy from non-carbohydrate sources such as fat).

Some food suggestions for KD includes eggs, avocado, fermented cheeses, seeds, nuts, butter, olive oil, fish, vegetables, vitamins, etc.

Ketone bodies are produced in response to KD which has several protective advantages. Multiple research works have shown that autophagy induced by starvation has neuro-protective advantages. For instance, the result of a study showed that rats fed with KD diets experienced a lesser amount of brain injury during a seizure.

3. Exercise. Exercise is one of the best stressors that are capable of triggering autophagy. One good thing about exercise according to reports from scientists is that it can trigger autophagy in many organs at the same time such as the liver, the muscles, the pancreas, the adipocytes, etc.[9]

Exercise helps the body regenerate and produce new tissues by breaking down worn out tissues and stimulating the body to create new ones. However, the amount of activity needed to stimulate autophagy is not yet clearly defined. For instance, 30 mins of exercise is enough to trigger autophagy in cardiac and skeletal muscles.

4. Sleep

Even though a vast majority of people replace rest time with binge-watching television, doing more work, and hanging out with friends, our body works at it's optimum when we acknowledge it's circadian rhythm or natural biological clock. This clock is in control of our sleeping cycles, as well as controls the process of autophagy.

It is vital to respect our circadian rhythm because it controls metabolic activities in the body. During our sleep, hormones are produced and released in our bodies. The absence of rest and sleep is seen as a stressful and distressing activity, and it negatively affects our health.

Sleep is therefore crucial in inducing autophagy as an absence of it alters the process of autophagy, and significantly slows it down.

Water-Fasting, Autophagy, and Anti-Aging – The Intersection

Aging is a result of a decrease in the rate and amount of autophagy, leading to accumulation of higher amounts of junks and cellular damage.

As organisms age, they experience a decrease in their autophagous capacities which means that they cannot service and repair themselves as they used to any longer. As a result of this, there'll be an accumulation of cell damage, and after some time (days or

---

[9] He, C., Sumpter, Jr., R., & Levine, B. (2012). Exercise induces autophagy in peripheral tissues and in the brain. *Autophagy, 8*(10), 1548-1551. doi: 10.4161/auto.21327

months or years), most of the cells become damaged or malfunctioning, losing their ability to function at an optimal level. If this degradation gets to vital organs, death becomes inevitably close.

Autophagy occurs in a cycle, fluctuating at different rates at different times of the day. An increased level of eating reduces autophagy, while fasting increases it.

Therefore, if the result of aging is a decreased rate of autophagy and an increase in damage accumulation, and the effect of fasting is an increased rate of autophagy, then fasting combats aging.

Anti-aging is the greatest significant benefit that comes with water fasting. Water fasting is, in fact, the most effective anti-aging strategy available. Therefore, anything that enhances autophagy can have anti-aging effects.

We won't enter a fasting state if we eat food every time, and will in principle, never speed up autophagy.

Remember, eating constantly, or "grazing" is a pro-aging activity, so, don't eat all the time.

Chapter 3: Myths and Symptoms of Water Fasting and Autophagy

Common Myths About Autophagy

There are lots of unknown facts about Autophagy – how it is measured, the mechanism of action, whether it is beneficial or not, and the effective quantity. There are also a lot of superstition and fabrications concerning autophagy.[10]

To begin Autophagy, you must fast for 3 to 5 days

To initiate autophagy, you must stimulate energy depletion and use up the body's own energy.

A person that eats a standard diet without cutting our protein or carbohydrates would have to fast for a minimum of 3 days to enter a ketotic state and initiate autophagy. Consequently, autophagy is controlled by maintaining stability between AMPK (or the AMP-activated protein kinase) and mTOR (or the mechanistic target of rapamycin).

You can certainly speed up the initiation of autophagy if you begin with lower energy stores, that is, you limit carbs and avoid overeating protein.

If your diet is based on whole foods, you are expected to enter the zone of therapy faster because there is a minimal quantity of excess energy in your body.

A 24-Hour Fast will give you Autophagy

Unfortunately, boosting autophagy is difficult when on a one-day fast unless you are doing lots of exercises while fasting.

Don't limit yourself to naïve the belief that you will enter autophagy if you fast for 16 hours because that is not a long enough timeframe. Some of the reasons why are:

---

[10] Land, S. (2019). Mistruths and Lies About Autophagy. Retrieved from https://siimland.com/mistruths-and-lies-about-autophagy/

- You must digest the nutrients from your last meal, so fasting is not initiated instantly

- After the absorption of nutrients, metabolism continues for four more hours after your food was eaten

- Foods like vegetables, fat, fiber and protein have a longer period of digestion.

You get into the state of fasting after 5 or 6 hours without eating because before this period, there is still food in your system, and you are using up calories from the previous food.

If your last meal was by 7 pm, your actual physiological fast does not start till midnight. So, if you are on a 16 or 20 hour fast, you have only spent 12 hours in a fasting state, which is not enough to initiate autophagy.

In addition to other hormonal advantages, Other benefits you would get are lowered inflammatory processes, reduced insulin. The appropriate period is 24 hours or more, as you would want to remain in the therapeutic zone for more than 2 hours.

More Autophagy is helpful

It would be beneficial to fast for at least 3 days to achieve meaningful autophagy. This will fight against tumors and malignancies and energize stem cells. Although, increased autophagy does not necessarily mean it would be helpful.

The harmful effects of excessive autophagy include:

- Excess autophagy might result in sarcopenia and muscle atrophy, which would, in turn, shorten your lifespan

- It makes tumor cells resistant to environmental stressors, making it harder for them to be killed.

- Autophagy promotes the replication of bacteria such as Brucella.

- ATG6/BECN1 which is the crucial gene for autophagy is a tumor suppressor. Although, in some cases, it might allow cancer to thrive by feeding it.

Although autophagy is incredible and it can help to improve your health, it is not always ideal. You would not want to always be in a state of autophagy throughout your life because there might be some side-effects that have not yet been discovered.

The best option is to alternate between autophagy and fasting- to practice extended fasts but not turn it into a do-or-die affair. We would not want to turn autophagy into a new diet ritual, right?

Starving is the same as Autophagy

From all that we have discussed, autophagy is not the same as starvation. You might think that fasting and going without food causes starvation, but that is a wrong approach to it.

Fasting results in starvation because you are not getting calories from food. Although, it would be almost impossible for the energy stores in your body to be completely depleted. These are the reasons:

- Autophagy degrades worn-out cells and proteins that will serve as an energy source again; when energy is insufficient, the body has no choice but to rechannel the less significant processes that won't take place when eating.

- You go into a ketotic state after fasting for several days. In a ketotic state, the main source of energy for the muscles and brain is ketones and fat. This alters everything because you would have to start using your biggest energy reserve- the adipose tissue. A car that uses up fuel after 100 miles might become starved, but a truck that has fuel stored in thousands of gallons can keep running for thousands of miles without hitting starvation. Remember, fat is the body's primary source of fuel.

- Everybody has at least some body fat. Body fat is a reservoir of energy that the body can survive on. People with as low as 10% of body fat have between 40 to 50,000 calories in "reserve." That is enough for weeks, even months.

- Simple autophagy lengthens lifespan and endurance. It is the primary cause of a longer life as observed in the restriction of calories.

In my point of view, autophagy and fasting are not the same as your body experiences the process of self-rejuvenation and restoration which does not happen when you eat. You might think it is starvation, but this is not correct. Even if you want to think of it as starvation, a small amount won't hurt; in fact, it is very beneficial to your health.

Autophagy develops your muscles

Developing your muscles without additional fuel or by going without food is extremely difficult because you need calories to build muscles.

Muscle development also requires the initiation of protein synthesis, which can only be done by eating protein. Fasting means that food is not the source of protein for your body, so your body is in a state of catabolism- break down, instead of anabolism-building up.

Hypothetically, autophagy also causes the degradation of worn-out proteins that are wandering about in your cells, and they are converted to synthesize proteins, but you still lack some specific amino acids such as leucine that are needed for protein synthesis in the muscle.

In a few cases, an overweight person that recently started resistance workouts may develop muscle while simultaneously losing fat. Although, it is mainly stimulated by the recent strength training.

Autophagy consumes flabby skin

It is believed that autophagy can consume excess skin that might be obvious after a recent weight loss and make it tighter. Although, there are some exceptions to this.

- Research conducted in 2014 in Japan discovered that old fibroblasts had reduced autophagy. Fibroblasts produce collagen in the skin, the cause of wrinkles and flabby skin.

- Another research conducted in Korea in 2018 discovered that old fibroblast has a higher rate of generating waste that then causes aging of the skin. The researchers concluded that autophagy is essential for reversing the process of aging by maintaining the health of the fibroblast.

Autophagy might help to reduce the rate at which the skin ages, but in reality, it does not consume flabby skin. It just promotes the processes that are responsible for the skin's elasticity and tightness.

In situations of excessive weight loss, autophagy and fasting can help to avoid excess flabby skin. You would certainly have some flabby skin after you have lost a lot of weight. Although, if your weight loss were achieved through fasting, there would be increased autophagy which would enable your skin to adjust to the new weight quickly.

Diets involving caloric restrictions in the absence of autophagy might generate a larger amount of flabby skin. Various studies have discovered that autophagy is vital to the functioning of the fibroblast and production of collagen.

Autophagy is not inhibited by fat

Though fat does not boost the levels of insulin as much as proteins or carbs, it would still make you feel full.

A ketotic state enhances macroautophagy of the brain through the activation of Sirt1 (also known as NAD-dependent deacetylase sirtuin-1). Ketone bodies promote intermediate autophagy that is aimed at some substrates and amino acids. Production of ketone bodies, including beta-hydroxybutyrate is increased during starvation and fasting, and they are also increased while on a ketogenic diet.

Although, mTOR reacts to all calories and not just glucose and amino acids. Additional energy from any source prevents autophagy.

Autophagy might not be completely inhibited by fat; it will reduce it to an extent. The quantity of fat that you consume determines if autophagy would be inhibited by fat. Small quantities of fat such as one tablespoon of MCT oil (concentrated medium chain fatty acids derived from coconut oil) might enhance intermediate autophagy due to an increase in the number of ketone bodies. Though, it is excessive once it exceeds 100 calories.

Autophagy is not inhibited by BCAAs

Amino acids are the major constituents of Branched-Chain Amino Acids, and it would certainly inhibit autophagy regardless of the quantity.

If you are in a ketotic state during your fast, and autophagy is stable, you should not be worried about muscle loss. Due to the increased ketone bodies, they both antagonize muscle catabolism.

Muscle is only lost if you move out of ketosis and quit autophagy without continuing with adequate protein and nutrients. The funny thing is that consuming BCAAs might result in that by tilting you towards a fed state and stopping ketosis.

Although it is not required, consuming BCAAs while fasting isn't so bad since you are using up glucose, hence, there is an increase in the level of blood glucose.

Consuming meat prevents autophagy

People believe that consuming meat or being on a protein-rich diet inhibits autophagy throughout your lifetime and speeds up the process of aging.

The essential factor in autophagy is the number of times you eat. It doesn't matter if you limit your meat and protein, once you eat three times in one day and do not fast for more than 24 hours, you might still not gain any relevant autophagy.

Additionally, autophagy is inhibited by insulin and carbohydrates so a vegan diet that is entirely based on plants would not cause autophagy too if you are eating too often.

Autophagy is not interrupted by fruits

The liver metabolizes fructose present in fruits and stores it as glycogen. Extra fructose is quickly changed into triglycerides. Autophagy is interrupted by fruits, and ketosis is stopped because it replenishes glycogen stores in the liver. Liver glycogen determines the balance between AMPK and mTOR. The liver acts as the primary center for energy metabolism and nutrient condition.

If you are eating only fruit with little or no fat or protein, you might remain in a state of catabolism, but it is not the same as autophagy. Autophagy is different from catabolism and loss of muscle. It is possible to be in extreme autophagy, and all your muscles are intact if you are in more extreme ketotic state and it is possible to lose a lot of muscle in the absence of autophagy.

Fruit is acceptable, and it is healthy in certain quantities. Although, it is not an ideal food that retains you in an autophagy every time.

Autophagy is inhibited by coffee

Autophagy is not inhibited by drinking coffee; neither will it break your fast. In reality, coffee enhances ketosis and autophagy.

Polyphenols present in coffee will promote autophagy on its own, though it is also enhanced by the drink via other methods. Caffeine stimulates lipolysis- the using up of fatty acids, this reduces insulin levels, enhances ketone bodies and increases AMPK

Black Coffee without cream, milk or sweeteners; which might increase insulin and inhibit the fast, promotes autophagy. Dairy and milk increase IGF-1 too that in turn makes mTOR active. Sweeteners with zero calorie increase insulin through the cephalic phase response that promotes insulin inside the gut.

It is risky to include MCT oil to your coffee; make sure it does not exceed one tablespoon.

It is impossible for autophagy to occur while eating

The truth is that the most efficient and certain way to start autophagy is to go without food and fast. Although there are some foods that enhance autophagy

They include

- Ginger which induces autophagy

- Medicinal mushroom induces autophagy

- Sulforaphane in cruciferous vegetables and broccoli speeds up autophagy

- Polyphenols from vegetables and dark berries induce autophagy

- Turmeric and Curcumin speeds up autophagy

- Resveratrol in grape skin, red wine, and dark berries speeds up autophagy

The precaution is that you might still need to limit your caloric intake mildly and you won't achieve the total benefits of autophagy.

These are only a few examples of some calorie containing foods that can enhance the process of autophagy

Autophagy is inhibited by exercise

Exercise is a great way to speed up autophagy. It initiates autophagy in the brain and peripheral tissues. Resistance workouts speed up mTOR signaling. Although not in the same manner as eating. Exercise only causes translocation of the mTOR complex nearer to the cell membrane and readies it for activation as soon as eating commences. Exercising implies that there is an increased sensitivity to mTOR activation, and it results in additional growth after work-out.

Also, long-term resistance workouts turn on autophagy and lower muscle apoptosis by regulating IGF-1 and its receptors.

After fasting, exercising is the closest activity that speeds up autophagy and enhances overall wellbeing. The most effective way is to do both and do them regularly.

Common Myths About Fasting

Next, this part disproves the common fallacies about snacking, the frequency of meals and fasting.

You will gain weight if you do not eat breakfast

The most important of the day is breakfast. There is a widespread misconception that there is something unique concerning breakfast.

Most people think that missing breakfast results in weight gain, cravings, and extreme hunger.

Though a lot of observational studies have discovered connections between not eating breakfast and obesity, this is because the person that typically skips breakfast is not very health conscious.

Although there might be some individual differences, it doesn't matter whether you eat breakfast.

However, kids who eat the first meal of the day have been found to be better at schoolwork. A few people have also achieved success with long-term weight loss indicating that they eat breakfast most times. This is one of those individual differences. For a few people, breakfast might be helpful while for others, it might not be.

Eating increases your metabolic rate

Consume a lot of small meals to continue the metabolic process. A lot of people think that eating additional meals results in higher metabolism, so your body depletes calories. The truth is, during the process of digestion and absorption of food, the body uses a particular quantity of energy. This is known as TEF(the thermic effect of food), and it is proportional to 0-3% fat, 5-10% carbs, and 20-30% protein.[11]

Usually, TEF is about 10% of the total quantity of consumed calories. Although, the important thing is not the frequency of your meals, but the number of calories consumed.

Consuming six meals with a calorie content of 600 gives the same benefit as eating three

[11] Westerterp, K. (2004). *Nutrition & Metabolism, 1*(1), 5. doi: 10.1186/1743-7075-1-5

meals with a calorie content of 1,000. In the two instances, the average thermic effect, which is 10% is 300 calories. This is evidenced by much feeding research in humans that have discovered that reducing or increasing the number of times you eat does not affect the calories used.[12]

Hunger is decreased by frequent eating

A few people think that snaking stops extreme hunger and cravings. However, a lot of research has studied this, and the outcomes are mixed. Though some research hypothesizes that frequent eating results in decreased hunger.

Further research discovered no benefits and some determined, elevated levels of hunger.[13][14]

One research compared six meals rich in protein to three other meals rich in protein, and it was discovered that the three meals were more effective for decreasing hunger.[15]

However, this is determined on an individual basis. If you experience a few cravings when you snack, you tend to binge-eat less; this might be a good idea.

There is no proof that eating or snacking decreases hunger for everybody.

Weight loss can be achieved with a lot of small meals

Eating frequent meals does not speed up the metabolic rate. It also does not decrease hunger.

If eating more meals does not affect the energy levels, then weight loss should not be affected. Science supports this. Most researches on this have discovered that the number of times you eat does not affect weight loss.[16]

For instance, research on 16 obese men and women did not discover any variation in

---

[12] Bellisle F, e. (2019). Meal frequency and energy balance. - PubMed - NCBI. Retrieved from https://www.ncbi.nlm.nih.gov/pubmed/9155494

[13] Smeets, A., & Westerterp-Plantenga, M. (2007). Acute effects on metabolism and appetite profile of one meal difference in the lower range of meal frequency. *British Journal Of Nutrition*, *99*(06). doi: 10.1017/s0007114507877646

[14] Leidy, H., Armstrong, C., Tang, M., Mattes, R., & Campbell, W. (2010). The Influence of Higher Protein Intake and Greater Eating Frequency on Appetite Control in Overweight and Obese Men. *Obesity*, *18*(9), 1725-1732. doi: 10.1038/oby.2010.45

[15] SPEECHLY, D., & BUFFENSTEIN, R. (1999). Greater Appetite Control Associated with an Increased Frequency of Eating in Lean Males. *Appetite*, *33*(3), 285-297. doi: 10.1006/appe.1999.0265

[16] Jon Schoenfeld, B., Albert Aragon, A., & Krieger, J. (2015). Effects of meal frequency on weight loss and body composition: a meta-analysis. *Nutrition Reviews*, *73*(2), 69-82. doi: 10.1093/nutrit/nuu017

appetite, weight, and loss of fat when contrasting three and six meals each day.[17]

Although if you discover that frequently eating makes it less hard to eat a few junk food and calories, maybe this would be beneficial to you.

For me, it is very stressful to eat frequently making it difficult to adhere to one healthy diet plan although it might be effective for some people.

The brain requires a steady supply of glucose

A few people think that if we do not consume carbs intermittently, our brain would be less active. The foundation of this is that the brain exclusively utilizes glucose as a source of energy. Although, what we often exclude is that the brain can effectively generate the glucose it requires via gluconeogenesis.

In a lot of cases, this might not be required because the body has a glycogen reservoir that can still supply the brain for a lot of hours.

While on a long-term fast, very low-carb diet or starvation can generate ketone bodies from dietary fats.

Ketone bodies generate energy for some of the brain decreasing the glucose needs greatly.

Thus, while on a long-term fast, the brain can still be sustained by consuming ketone bodies and glucose generated from fats and protein. From the history of evolution, it is pointless to think that we would not be able to live in the absence of a steady source of carbohydrates. If this were truly the case, then humans would have gone into extinction since.

Although a few people say that they experience hypoglycemia after going without food. If this happens to you, you should probably adhere to eating more meals, or confirm from your doctor before you make changes.

It is healthy to snack and eat frequently

The body cannot naturally remain in a fed state. During human evolution, we had to bear times of food shortages. This is proof that fasting for a short period initiates a

---

[17] Cameron, J., Cyr, M., & Doucet, É. (2009). Increased meal frequency does not promote greater weight loss in subjects who were prescribed an 8-week equi-energetic energy-restricted diet. *British Journal Of Nutrition*, 1. doi: 10.1017/s0007114509992984

process of cell repair known as autophagy where the cells utilize workout and malfunctioning proteins as a source of fuel. Autophagy can prevent aging and diseases such as Alzheimer's disease; it may even decrease the risk of cancer. Fasting at various times is very beneficial to metabolism.[18]

Also, some researchers have proposed that snacking and frequent eating can otherwise affect your health and increase the risk of diseases.

For instance, one research discovered that a diet that involves frequent eating and high amounts of calories could increase the risk of a fatty liver.[19]

Some observational studies have also discovered that people that eat frequently have an increased risk of colorectal cancer.[20]

Fasting makes your body go into starvation

The general thoughts concerning fasting at intervals are that it might tilt your body into a period of starvation, basically called adaptive thermogenesis. This can result in burning up fewer quantities of calories each day. Although this occurs with losing weight, irrespective of the strategy used. There is no proof that this is more common with intermittent fasting compared with other methods of weight loss.

There is proof that fasting for short-term increases metabolism. This is because of a sudden increase in noradrenaline (norepinephrine) which activates fat cells to degrade body fat and enhance the metabolic rate.

Research has discovered that fasting for about 48 hours can improve metabolic rate three times faster, although if you fast for a longer period, this can be modified, and the metabolic rate can be further reduced than the standard rate.

One research discovered that fasting at least once in 22 days did not result in a reduction in metabolism, but the subjects lost 4% of their body fat which is excellent for less than three weeks of fasting.[21]

---

[18] Alirezaei, M., Kemball, C., Flynn, C., Wood, M., Whitton, J., & Kiosses, W. (2010). Short-term fasting induces profound neuronal autophagy. *Autophagy, 6*(6), 702-710. doi: 10.4161/auto.6.6.12376

[19] Koopman, K., Caan, M., Nederveen, A., Pels, A., Ackermans, M., & Fliers, E. et al. (2014). Hypercaloric diets with increased meal frequency, but not meal size, increase intrahepatic triglycerides: A randomized controlled trial. *Hepatology, 60*(2), 545-553. doi: 10.1002/hep.27149

[20] de Verdier, M., & Longnecker, M. (1992). Eating frequency—a neglected risk factor for colon cancer?. *Cancer Causes & Control, 3*(1), 77-81. doi: 10.1007/bf00051916

[21] Heilbronn, L., Smith, S., Martin, C., Anton, S., & Ravussin, E. (2005). Alternate-day fasting in nonobese subjects: effects on body weight, body composition, and energy metabolism. *The American Journal Of Clinical Nutrition, 81*(1), 69-73. doi: 10.1093/ajcn/81.1.69

There is a minimum amount of protein that can be utilized for every meal

Some people say that for every meal, only 30 grams of protein is digested and that we should eat meals every 2 or 3 hours to optimize muscle gain.

Although science does not back this up, research has shown that there is no obvious variation in muscle mass if you consume protein more frequently.[22] The overall quantity of protein consumed the most significant factor for most people, not the frequency of meals that contains protein.

You lose muscle when you undergo intermittent fasting

A few people think that fasting uses up muscles as an energy source.

Generally, this occurs when we diet, but there is no proof that this occurs with intermittent fasting compared to other strategies. Some researchers have proposed that intermittent fasting can effectively maintain muscle mass. Review research discovered that intermittent calorie limitation resulted in the same degree of weight loss seen in continuous calorie limitation but more decrease in muscle mass.[23]

Another research also involved the subject eating the same quantity of calories that they usually eat, with the exclusion of one large meal in the evening.[24]

The subjects lost body fat and had a fare increase (close to statistical significance) in their muscle mass, together with a lot of other benefits on the health.

A lot of bodybuilders also adopt intermittent fasting since it effectively maintains a large quantity of muscle with a reduced percentage of body fat.

It is unhealthy to carry out Intermittent Fasting

A few people assume that fasting might be hazardous, but this is nowhere close to the truth.

---

[22] Arnal, M., Mosoni, L., Boirie, Y., Houlier, M., Morin, L., & Verdier, E. et al. (1999). Protein pulse feeding improves protein retention in elderly women. *The American Journal Of Clinical Nutrition, 69*(6), 1202-1208. doi: 10.1093/ajcn/69.6.1202

[23] Varady, K. (2011). Intermittent versus daily calorie restriction: which diet regimen is more effective for weight loss?. *Obesity Reviews, 12*(7), e593-e601. doi: 10.1111/j.1467-789x.2011.00873.x

[24] Stote, K., Baer, D., Spears, K., Paul, D., Harris, G., & Rumpler, W. et al. (2007). A controlled trial of reduced meal frequency without caloric restriction in healthy, normal-weight, middle-aged adults. *The American Journal Of Clinical Nutrition, 85*(4), 981-988. doi: 10.1093/ajcn/85.4.981

For instance, intermittent fasting alters the expression of genes that increase lifespan and prevent some diseases, and it has been discovered to increase the lifespan of tested animals. It is also very significant to metabolism, like enhanced sensitivity to insulin, and a decrease in different risk factors for heart diseases.

Also, it might be beneficial to mental health by increasing the levels of hormones known as BDNF (brain-derived neurotrophic factor). This may also prevent depression and other brain disorders.

You eat a lot while fasting intermittently

A few people say that intermittent fasting would not result in weight loss, because it makes you overeat. This might be true. People are likely to eat more food while fasting compared periods of not fasting. This means that they try to replace the calories that were lost while fasting by increased eating over the subsequent meals.

Although, this replacement is incomplete. A research discovered that people who went without food for an entire day ate an additional 500 calories the following day. So, they used up 2,400 calories on the days they fasted then replaced with 500 calories the following day. The overall decrease in calorie consumption was 1,900 calories which is quite a huge loss for just two days.[25]

Intermittent fasting lowers total food insulin and enhances metabolic rate. It lowers the levels of insulin, raises norepinephrine and enhances growth hormones in humans five times. As a result of these factors, intermittent fasting causes fat loss instead of gain. Review research conducted in 2014 discovered that fasting for 3-24 weeks resulted in a 4-7% reduction in stomach fat and weight loss of 3-8%. In this research, intermittent fasting resulted in a weight loss of 0.55 pound every week, compared to intermittent fasting that resulted in 1.65 pounds weight loss every week. In reality, intermittent fasting is the strongest strategy for weight loss worldwide. It is not at all true to say that it causes you to overeat and enter starvation mode and eventual weight gain.

Symptoms of Water Fasting

At the beginning of water fast you might notice a lot of beneficial effects and some side-

---

[25] Barnosky, A., Hoddy, K., Unterman, T., & Varady, K. (2014). Intermittent fasting vs daily calorie restriction for type 2 diabetes prevention: a review of human findings. *Translational Research, 164*(4), 302-311. doi: 10.1016/j.trsl.2014.05.013

effects. This is to be expected. We will be discussing these so that you can have a deeper knowledge of what your body is going through.

These symptoms are to be expected and should not cause any worry[26]

Hunger. This is caused by ghrelin secreted by the stomach as a reaction to an empty stomach or as an automatic secretion at the times when we usually feed. Do not be concerned; you won't die; neither are you starving; this is just a response to physiological hormones in your body.

Fatigue. This happens because the body has not fully adjusted to using ketones and fat as a source of energy.

Changes in mood. While the body is adjusting to the use of fat in place of sugar, the brain might be hypoglycemic at times, and this can cause brain haziness, depression, mental weakness, and irritability. You might feel headaches too.

Mental Weakness. We have adapted to our brain having a constant supply of sugar as an energy source; this low level of sugar generates less energy for the brain. Also, neurotransmitters are stimulated by the presence of food, so the levels decrease. If you are used to a ketogenic diet, you might not experience a lot of mental weakness on the first day.

Sleep Disturbances. For a few people, the fast makes them sleep peacefully while it is difficult for others. The more experienced you are with the ketogenic diet, the less hypoglycemia you will feel and you will observe a more peaceful sleep. It can be very beneficial to enhance your sleep with melatonin, adaptogenic spices such as ashwagandha, additional magnesium, and L-theanine as well.

Cravings. The brain responds to emotional feelings through cravings. Eating stimulates excitatory brain neurotransmitters like serotonin and dopamine. Generally, this is very good since eating is enjoyable. Fasting makes our brain too dependent on these feelings, and it causes an increase in the signals that would be sent to satisfy these feelings.

Rashes. You might probably experience rashes during your fast. Rashes happen in 10% of people, and the rashes are as a result of alterations in the skin microflora. Fasting reduces this microflora and a lot of harmful chemicals are released into the circulatory system and causes release Substance P and histamine in the skin that results in inflammation and rashes. They will fade eventually and are symptoms of a response to healing

---

[26] 5 Day Water Fast: What to Expect on the Healing Journey - DrJockers.com. (2019). Retrieved from https://drjockers.com/water-fast/

Frequent urination. When the body degrades glycogen into energy, it also causes a release of water into the urinary system. Frequent urination is an expected response. You should also drink additional water than you normally drink and this will increase the quantity of your urine.

Tongue Changes. Your tongue might become black, white or yellow. This color change should be expected as part of the body's physiological detoxification.

Cold. When there is a sensation of food shortage by the body, the body starts to reduce the production of active thyroid hormone. This reduction helps to enhance the use of energy in the body, and the usual symptom is developing cold extremities and coldness all over the body.

When Should You Stop the Fast?

On the fourth day, you should have adapted, and it is simpler to continue the fast for longer if desired. Remember, some people who have disorders in metabolism or extreme stress might have some problems and might have to stop the fast early. These are the red flags you should look out for:

Excruciating Pain. If you experience excruciating pain while fasting, then stop the fast.

Increased loss of hair. Once you observe hair loss in chunks, stop the fast.

Extreme Hunger. You might experience a mild desire for food, but you should not feel actual hunger. If you feel this symptom, listen to your body and stop the fast.

Extreme Weight Loss. If you feel or look gaunt and tired, then stop the fast.

Loss of consciousness and fainting. If you experience loss of consciousness and faint, or you feel very dizzy, break the fast.

Palpitations. If you are experiencing heart palpitations that are making you worried or affecting your sleep, stop the fast.

Intense Vomiting or Diarrhea. This could result in the loss of excess electrolytes, and you should stop the fast.

You should not be embarrassed about breaking your fast early. The body becomes healthier and stronger after subsequent fasts. If you are experiencing major health issues, then you should engage in the water fast every 1-3 months, and eventually, you will experience a reduction in these stressful symptoms, and you would be able to fast for five whole days effortlessly.

Chapter 4: Starting a Water Fast

Common Kinds of Water Fasting:

Intermittent Water Fasting. There are distinct periods in each day for eating and fasting. This has an effect of limiting your daily eating window to predetermined hours, and it usually lasts for 8 to 24 hours.

Extended Fast. Extending your fast is a better way of burning body fat as it involves water fasting for a couple of days at a stretch. With prolonged fasting, the longer the fast, the more beneficial the process.

- 3-day water fast. You avoid eating food for 72 hours.

- 7 – 10-day water fast. The average time required to reach ketosis is roughly 72 hours. Therefore, you'll spend approximately 48 hours in ketosis

- 14 – 40-day water fast. In mental and physical terms, this is quite challenging. It is best suited for deeper healings.

Intermittent Fasting

Intermittent fasting (IF) is essentially an eating pattern whereby you alternate between periods of eating and fasting. Here, the time of eventual consumption of food is what is specified. The characteristics as mentioned above make it less of a diet and more of an eating pattern. Daily 16 hour fasts or fasting for 24 hours, twice a week are conventional intermittent fasting methods.

The act of fasting is one that has been evident in every stage of human evolution. For example, the hunter-gatherers of old did not have the means to preserve food as we do now neither was food available all year round. Since food was in short supply, humans evolved and gained the ability to live without food for extended periods.

As a matter of fact, intermittent fasting is a practice that is closer to our natural tendencies than eating 3 or more meals per day.

Intermittent fasting is usually used as a precursor to water fasting. It helps you ease into water fasting.

There are several intermittent fasting methods in existence, and they all have varying levels of effectiveness based on an individual's needs. Among the intermittent fasting methods, six methods are the most common. They are:

1. The 16/8 Method: Fast for 16 hours each day

When utilizing the method, you fast for 14 – 16 hours daily. This method restricts your eating window to 8-10 hours, during which you can have 2 or more meals. Popularized by fitness expert Martin Berkhan, the 16/8 method is also called the Leangains protocol.

The most common form of this method that produces the most success is by eating dinner and skipping breakfast the following day. In a scenario where your last meal was around 8 pm, and you don't eat until noon the following day, the fasting period is more or less 16 hours.

Women have been observed to perform better on slightly shorter fasts, so it is recommended that they fast for 14-15 hours. This method can be complicated initially for individuals that get hungry in the morning. Breakfast skippers, on the other hand, eat this way instinctively.

To help reduce hunger levels during the fast, you can drink coffee, non-caloric beverages, and water. Doing this helps with the transition to water fast.

In general, you should avoid junk foods or excessive amounts of calories during your eating window as eating such food items undermine the purpose of the fast. You should eat healthy foods.

2. The 5:2 Diet: Fast for two days per week.

This diet involves regularly eating for all but two days a week and is also referred to as the Fast Diet. On two selected days, calories consumed should be restricted to 500-600 calories on each day. For women, the recommended calorie intake is 500 calories while for men it's 600 calories. An example of this can involve eating normally on all days except Mondays and Thursdays, where you eat two small meals (300 calories per meal for men and 250 calories for women).

3. Eat-Stop-Eat: Do a 24-hour fast, once or twice a week

Here, a 24-hour fast is carried out once or twice a week. An example of this method is eating dinner on Monday at 7 pm and fasting until 7 pm the following day.

This method is not only limited to dinner to dinner cycles, but it can also be from breakfast one day to breakfast the following day and lunch to lunch. All cycles achieve the same result. Solid food is not allowed, but you can drink water, coffee, and non-caloric beverages.

You have to eat appropriately during eating periods while utilizing this method as a means of losing weight.

The downside to this method is the difficulty of a 24 hour fast for a lot of people. It is better to start from 14-16 hours fast and gradually work your way up to 24 hours fast.

4. Alternate Day Fasting: Fast every other day.

The alternate day fast is a full fast where you fast one day and eat the other day properly, i.e., you fast every other day. There are many variations of this method, and some of them have an allowance of 500 calories on fasting days.

Given the difficulty of a full fast every other day, I wouldn't recommend this variant for beginners.

This method is unpleasant and generally unsustainable in the long term because you will go to bed hungry several times in a given week.

5. The Warrior Diet: Fast during the day, eat a huge meal at night.

Here, you eat a small proportion of raw vegetables and fruits during the day. At night, you eat a substantial meal within a 4-hour eating window.

One of the first popular diets to incorporate intermittent fasting; the Warrior diet has similar food choices which are similar to a paleo diet- whole, unprocessed foods that are similar to the form in which they exist in nature.

Due to the large caloric intake involved, this isn't recommended during water fasting.

6. Spontaneous Meal Skipping: Skip meals when convenient.

Here, a strict intermittent fasting plan is not necessary for you to reap certain benefits of the fast. You can also skip meals when you are too busy to make a meal or when you are not hungry.

''People needing to eat every few hours to prevent themselves from losing muscle as a result of starvation" is a myth. Our bodies have what it takes to endure extended periods without food.

Using this method is as simple as skipping a meal if you are not hungry and eating healthy foods for subsequent meals. It can also involve carrying out a short fast while traveling. As long as you are skipping 1 or 2 meals, you are carrying out a spontaneous intermittent fast.

Extended Fasting

This can be embarked upon after about two weeks of intermittent fasting and/or ketogenic diet.

The three-day water fast

The three-day water fast is the most essential fast as three days is the period when your body's healing metabolism is unlocked. Three-day fasts also serve as stepping stones essential to moving on to longer fasts in which you undergo the deepest healing. Water fasting of any length can be made easier if you practice three-day fasts regularly.

At first, the three-day fast is the hardest of all fasts, and it is essential that you follow all the steps required for you to increase your chances of having a smooth experience.

Given its difficulty and excessive body demands, you must be comfortable with intermittent fasting before you can move on to the three-day fast.

As a beginner, the majority of the challenges of the three-day fast are physical because your body must learn to enter a state of ketosis.

So, let's look at what happens over these three days and their accompanying feelings.

Day 1: You will slowly deplete your carbohydrate reserves (glycogen) stored in your liver and the tissues surrounding your muscles on the first day. This won't be a challenge for you physiologically as you are familiar with the experience of surviving without food for a day. An extension of going without food for a day is going without food for three days, and this should enable you to focus on the physical changes occurring within you. Over these three days, you will often find yourself face to face with your ego in that you will face your addictions to food rather than giving in to the existential fear of survival presented by your ego.

Day 2: Your glycogen reserves will run out by the beginning of the second day. When you get to this point, your experience with fasting determines how you feel. Generally, you'll feel great because as your glycogen stores run out, your body will initiate ketosis. At this time, you will not suffer "loss of power."

Things will go differently if your body hasn't adapted to ketosis. In this scenario, after your glycogen reserves are depleted, your body will quickly search for an alternative energy source. Since your body hasn't learned to access the metabolic pathways that lead to the burning of fat through ketosis, it'll move to the closest source of energy: burning protein. The protein in question is your muscle tissue. However, you will not lose a significant portion of your muscle mass, probably just a few hundred grams, and this is until your body perfects ketosis usually by the end of the third day. At that point, any additional loss of muscle mass is negligible.

Around this time, you will feel weak, and this is a result of the relatively low levels of energy within you. As a result of burning through protein present in muscle tissue, you may experience aches in your back and leg muscles. The lack of energy and the low blood sugar levels contribute to the headaches you may experience during this period. The onset of detoxification can also contribute to this. You may feel dull aches around your kidneys as they work above their usual levels. This overwork is caused by the excessive amount of detoxification that the kidneys have to carry out to cope with the influx of toxins coming from the metabolism of proteins and fat cells. If you experience such symptoms, it's advisable to ensure you are getting enough fluids: at least a quart/liter or two per day. As there is no fixed minimal limit of the number of fluids you are required to drink, it becomes dependent on a person's level of toxicity. You should drink more if you have a high toxicity level. You should also reduce fluid intake if you have a low toxicity level. A lot of people can drink as much as 3-4 quarts/liters a day.

Be ready to feel awful while going through your initial three-day fasts. However, the "awful" feelings of general lack of energy and aches are very similar to what you experience when you have the flu and those times are usually bearable. You don't need to worry, neither do you need to give up at the point because you'll survive, and all these symptoms will pass.

Day 3: In terms of physiological processes, the third day is a continuation of the second day. In most cases, you feel at your worst at the end of the second day. You may also be at your lowest at the beginning of the third day. As the switch to ketosis approaches completion, things will begin to improve in terms of how you feel.

You'll probably be emotionally and physically drained after your first few three-day fasts. At the end of the third day, you don't need to do anything more as you would have accomplished your mission. After your first three-day fasts, you would have awakened your body's healing metabolism, and this will make subsequent fasts easier. Another thing you would have achieved is a significant degree of detoxification. Once your body has fully acclimatized to the three-day fast, you should take on a longer, more cleansing fast.

On getting to the end of the third day, you can reward yourself with freshly squeezed orange juice. As opposed to long fasts, there's no need for a long transition back to eating after the fast. It is important to note that the first few meals before and after the fast should be light: mostly fruits and vegetables. You shouldn't give in to your ego and eat too much. You should avoid this temptation and follow your healthy appetite. You would have undergone a few changes: your stomach would have shrunk, and your digestive system would have slowed down significantly. The direct result of this is that you need a few days to get things back to their optimum levels. If you honestly follow our appetite, you'll begin to eat normally in a few days.

The 7 – 10-day Water Fast

The best time to advance to this type of extended fast is when you are comfortable with the three-day fast, and your body can easily transit into a state of ketosis. You can only enjoy the full benefits of detoxification when your body begins to draw energy solely from your fat cells. The implication of this is a three-day fast is not enough to tackle the deeper issues that need healing.

The thought of undergoing a 7-10 day fast would be daunting especially if you struggled with your first few three-day fasts. Attending a fasting retreat is very helpful to gain the deepest experience from your fast.

7-10-day fasts are not as emotionally and physically demanding as you expect, and this is surely the case if you're healthy and don't have serious issues when you undergo detox. What makes the fast easier than it seems is because your body does the most difficult part of the work, which is the establishment of ketosis, during the first three days. The efficiency at which ketosis occurs increases significantly after the third day. The result of this increased efficiency is that you feel better overall and you have more energy at your disposal. As days progress, the fast feels like a celebration of the freedom you have gained over the daily need to eat food. A clearer consciousness usually accompanies this freedom, and a lighter body and these feel so good that a lot of people feel reluctant to go back to eating food after the fast. There's a significant degree of purity that comes with being able to live without the needs and addictions of food distracting you.

Let's take a look at how you will feel as you go through stages of 7-10-day water fast:

Days 1-3: The first three days of a 7-10 day fast are more or less the same as the entirety of a three day fast. As you gain experience, this part becomes easier and even enjoyable. Your body's ability to undergo ketosis will improve immensely over time.

Days 4-6: Your body will begin to heal and carry out detoxification once you fully enter ketosis. Certain symptoms will make you aware of the stage: your breath, general body odor, and even your sweat will begin to stink. This occurs because your body expels toxins through your skin. As a result of these physiological stages, you may want to avoid frequent social interactions. The upside to this is as you witness your body expelling such repulsive things, it makes you appreciate the fact that you have gotten rid of them. This also gives you the willpower to take up fasting again in the future; even it was hard for you in the beginning. To reap the full benefits, you should convert to water fasting on the fourth or fifth day of your first 7-10 day fast - especially when your tongue produces an unpleasant metallic tasting froth.

The detoxification can place a significant burden on the kidneys and muscles, causing them to ache. Fortunately, the pain is usually a lot more bearable at this stage compared to the first three days. It is harder during the first three days because you are low on energy at that stage. There will be periods where you will have a clear consciousness and feel great physically. Alternatively, you will also notice periods where you are weaker and heavier. Such periods are periods of deeper cleansing. Things change a lot during longer fasts. Things change from hour to hour, from day to day and the sequences do not follow any inherent logic. As such, in-depth analysis is of no use. You simply have to trust your body to know where to heal, how and what to detox and when to rest in between the more intensive segments of the fast.

Days 7-10: It's okay to undergo four- or five-day fasts. The benefits of fasting generally increase with every additional day of fasting. However, you should only extend your fast to the 7-10 part if you are emotionally ready to move beyond a three day fast. At this stage, you experience what is called a '' healing crisis". This is a state where your body advances from basic detox and begins to uncover and heal deeper injuries, traumas, and illnesses.

A healing crisis will resemble a returning illness that is intensified during the fast. If you don't understand what's going on, you may be worried. The truth is everything you are going through at this point is perfectly normal. What occurs within your body at the point is this: the fasting procedure forces a deep-lying illness out of your body's physical depths and/or the subconscious of your mind. Its symptoms temporarily accompany the resurfacing of the said illness although they may be more acute than before. This may be an uncomfortable experience, but it is necessary to bring forth these illnesses to ensure your body heals and permanently expels them. This level of healing is unachievable using western medicine because toxic (allopathic) drugs and physical procedures simply suppress symptoms. This is not the same as dealing with the root causes of a given illness.

Extended Healing Fasts(14-40 days)

It seems surprising that fasting for two weeks or more is even a thing, right?

The proportion of people in the western world that will ever undertake an extended fast of 14 days or more is even smaller than the minuscule proportion of people in the western world that carry out a water fast. The reason for this? There is no need as occasional 7-10-day fasts accompanied by regular short fasts are enough to keep you healthy.

The deepest forms of healing can only be assessed through such long fasts as the extended fast. This healing can cure even the most serious illnesses deemed incurable by Western medicine. Contrary to what allopathic doctors tell you, conditions like chronic high blood pressure, multiple sclerosis, Type II diabetes, certain types of tumors as well as autoimmune disorders are all curable. They can be permanently healed through water fasting.

Only through extending the length of our fast can we experience the deepest spiritual cleansing. A reference point nowadays is the biblical 40-day fasts of Moses and Jesus even though other religions have demanded 40-day water fasts. It is said that even Pythagoras required potential students to carry out a 40 day fast as a prerequisite for his acceptance. We tend to dislike the idea of giving up food for an extended period; in actuality, it is just a matter of our unwillingness to forgo the pleasures and addictions of life. You shouldn't give in to the voices in your head that tell you that you will starve to death. As long as you are not severely malnourished and underweight, you have around 100,000 calories on you. The calories are trapped deep within your fat tissue, and they can only be released by ketosis. These calories are more than enough to last you for 40 days. You are able to even fast for much longer than 40 days if you are overweight even though this is not advisable.

On a basic level, the idea of an extended fast continues the process of the 7-10 day fast. The key difference is the extended fast is more powerful when it comes to the healing process associated with it which in this case, is the "healing crisis". A healing crisis initially occurs around the end of the first week of water fasting. It is characterized by the resurgence of symptoms of old traumas, illnesses and injuries before the afflictions in question are permanently expelled from the body. An identical process occurs at the end of the second week of water fasting, and this process is the main driving force behind the decision to extend a 7-10 day fast to make it at least 14 days. This process is the second healing crisis, and it causes even deeper issues that the first healing crisis couldn't reach. It heals and permanently expels any issues left from the first healing crisis. The meaning of all this is your body begins to tackle the more serious health issues from the beginning of the second week of water fasting. Before this point, your body has been removing the toxins that accumulated from everyday living especially for an individual that doesn't fast regularly.

At times, the most serious as well as the deepest health issues need healing crises that occur much later in the fast. "Much later " in this case can be 20, 30 or 40 days as there is no accurate way of predicting the time of its occurrence. You just have to trust your body as well as nature.

At times, healing will occur without a serious healing crisis. In cases like these, the symptoms of trauma or illness will abruptly vanish. When this happens, it's a sign that you have gotten rid of a health issue. Continuing the fast and knowing the best time to end the fast at this point is difficult. Situations like these give rise to the need for medical supervision while conducting an extended fast. Working with a professional also ensures you don't go beyond your body's nutritional capabilities while fasting.

Unless you feel there is a serious health issue buried within your body or you have a desire to reach your spiritual depths, there is no need for a fast exceeding the 7-10 day fast since a significant amount of healing and detox occurs during such a fast. For a healthy lifestyle, all you need are weekly 24- or 36-hour fasts (or regular intermittent fasting instead) combined with a 7-10 day fast from time to time. The frequency with which you undertake a 7-10 day fast is at your discretion. However, you shouldn't force your body to undergo such stress before it is ready even if you strongly feel it is the right thing to do. You can begin to trust your body once it has grown accustomed to the rigors of a 1-3 day fast because your body will know exactly what is best for you at this point. In fact, you will know when the time is right because you will feel an inner urge to do a 7-10 day fast and you will look forward to it. This urge comes once in a few years for some individuals while for some, it can come more than once in a given year. You just need to "listen" to your body.

There is a risk of a fast turning to starvation if you extend it indefinitely and this is a line you should never cross! At the point of starvation when even your fat stores are depleted, your body begins to break down your muscle tissue and internal organs. This can cause serious damage to you. The good thing is, your body will send you a very clear sign before any serious damage is done: extreme hunger. Two other scenarios should prompt you to end a fast. The first is a scenario whereby you deplete your muscle tissue before you deplete your fat reserves. Although ketosis is a very efficient process, it does not provide glucose which is essential as a fuel for the brain. Therefore, the glucose which can't be gotten from fat metabolism must be gotten from the depletion of muscles. The second scenario/ possibility is one where you run out of electrolytes (blood salts. This is a very dangerous situation to be in even though it is very unlikely. To prevent this scenario, you should get your blood tested at regular intervals after the initial 7 -10 days of fasting.

Variations of Water Fasting

The following are some of the most common ways to do an extended fast.

- **Strict Water Fasting.** Here, you only drink water, usually for several days in a row (typically no less than 24 hours).

- **Water plus non-caloric beverages.** This is a slight variation of water fast. In addition to drinking water, you can drink other non- caloric beverages like herbal tea and coffee (without milk, sugar or other sweeteners, including artificial non-caloric sweeteners).

- **Bone broth variation.** In this variation, you are allowed to consume a bone broth. A bone broth contains healthy fats and a lot of proteins, so this fast is not considered a true fast.

To experience good results, you can take bone broth, water as well as coffee and tea. If doing this provides results that you feel are desirable, you should continue the variant of the extended fast. "If you begin to get poor results with a bone broth or fat fasting, you can go to classic water-only fast."

- **Fat Fasting.** In this variant, you add healthy fats such as bulletproof coffee (black coffee with butter, coconut oil or MCT oil) in addition to water and non-caloric beverages. You also simply add the fat to your tea.

Chapter 5: Transitioning from a Regular Diet to Fasting

You can do a water fast if you are one of those people who eat until they are full one day and then easily avoid eating the following day. You don't need to plan it. However, you need to make plans for a smart transition into your next water fast if you are an individual who ends up eating an excessive amount of unhealthy food after a couple of days (or even hours) into your water fast.

Taking your time to plan and prepare for a water fast will greatly improve your chances of seeing the fast through till the end.

You need to get used to the idea of fasting before you start the real thing. Doing this enables you to transition to your next water fast properly.

You will discover that the fasting experience is a whole lot easier when you carry out a proper transition into full-blown water fast, you are also more likely to complete the required duration of the fast.

Reducing the size of your meals before you begin the fast is a major step in preparing yourself for a water fast.

You should eat most vegetables and fruits before beginning your fast. You should also eradicate processed foods, sugar and caffeine from your diet at least 2-3 days before your intended fast.

Before you begin your water fast, you should gradually reduce your portion sizes weeks before the commencement of your water fast. It is best if you do this at least a couple of days before you begin.

Intermittent fasting is also useful in making the transition to full water fast.

This can be simple as initially skipping food until noon every day. You will begin to skip food to 5 PM as you get closer to your fast. The time of your first meal will be at 7 PM and so on.

For someone who hasn't done a water fast before, this will provide you with a very good insight into the way things will be when you begin your water fast.

You might want to make a few adjustments before you begin water fast, especially if you find it difficult to stay away from food till 7 PM.

By the time of you get comfortable with the idea of skipping meals till 7 PM, your stomach, as well as your mind, are fully prepared to go completely without food.

It is possible to have a plan that is spread out over a month:

- Week 1: Skip breakfast
- Week 2: Skip both breakfast and lunch
- Week 3: Skip breakfast and lunch. You will also begin to decrease your dinner portions
- Week 4: Begin your water fast

What to Eat During the Transition Over to Water-Fasting

After the establishment of your healing metabolism, your digestive system will just have finished shutting down its day to day functions. Due to the temporary change, the majority of hunger pangs will begin to reduce in intensity after this point. Since your digestion has, in essence, come to a halt, it becomes very important for you to contemplate what and how you eat during the transition period before and after any fast that goes beyond three days.

To prevent your digestive system from shutting down with food being present in the intestines, you must ensure a proper transition to a fast. If the transition is not done properly, the remaining food will rot, and that is as uncomfortable as it sounds. The toxic by-products liberated from rotting food are detrimental to the body.

You will need to begin to change your eating habits around two or three weeks before the water fasting, and this is aimed at enhancing your nutrient uptake and familiarizing yourself with a healthy water fast.

- **Say goodbye to:** fast food, white flours, processed junk foods, processed meats, diet soda and drinks including regular soda, artificially and sugar-sweetened beverages and alcohol. You should also begin to keep off caffeine.
- **Say hello to:** Fresh juice with a variety of fruits and vegetables, salads, smoothies, soups as well as seeds, whole grains, natural nut butter, nuts, legumes, and beans. You should get used to drinking more water and enjoying the benefits of staying hydrated. Try to increase your water intake to 64 oz (2l) of water per day and add fresh orange, lemon or lime for flavor and vitamin C

- **Transition off animal proteins:** you should choose wild fish when possible as well as organic/pasture-raised eggs and reduce poultry consumption gradually during the week. If you are going to eat red meat, ensure it is lean, grass-fed, and don't eat beyond day 3 of the transition week.

- **Transition off dairy:** Ensure you choose organic dairy without added sugars For non-dairy milk like almond, make sure it is unsweetened. Gradually make the transition from cow's cheese to goat cheese once you get to the middle of the week. By the end of day 5, dairy should no longer be a part of your diet.

What to Drink During Fasting Without Breaking the Fast?

When engaging in water fasting, try to avoid all forms of caloric intake for some time. You're not supposed to eat food, desserts or snacks or even drink juices.

DUH! - It's a period where we starve!

At the point your body goes into a fasted state, your physiology changes into mild ketosis, which adds to fat burning and minimizes appetite. That is, the more you fast, the deeper you get into ketosis, it becomes easier.

However, we still have some additional beverages you can consume while fasting and won't end the fast. Factually, these beverages work to enhance the effectiveness of your fast as they empower cellular detoxification, cleansing of your gut and ketosis. What do you think is best to eat or drink while fasting?

Baking Soda. Although most people only use baking soda for cooking, it also has numerous health benefits unknown to many.

- It works for digestive problems

- It relieves bloating and constipation

- It helps to eliminate bad bacteria and parasites

- Lessens muscle soreness and fatigue

- Makes the acidity in the gut ineffective

- Enables the balance of pH levels available in the body

A teaspoon of baking could be added to your water for consumption to enhance physical performance and total well-being.

During the period of water-fasting, it is advisable to watch over your electrolytes because you tend to relieve yourself of minerals and water.

Baking soda contains 100% sodium bicarbonate, which is necessary to achieve some amount of sodium during fasting but, to be frank, it has an awful taste, so it is best used to curb hunger. Thankfully, after drinking it, you won't be left with an aftertaste, and you should be able to continue with your fast easier.

Glauber's Salts. When you aim to engage in water fasting for health reasons and to encourage cellular cleansing, then look into consuming Glauber's salt.

Glauber's salt serves as a mild laxative that activates bowel movements. By adding 5-20 grams of Glauber's salt into water, constipation can be eliminated, bloating can be minimized, and the digestive tract is left clean. Adding more to this amount could lead to diarrhea and can also cause dehydration, so remember not to overuse it.

Herbal Teas. Herbal teas have a wonderful taste and try to use it to stave off hunger during water fasting. As a bonus, they possess some detoxifying and various medicinal benefits as well.

- Chamomile helps to calm a worrying stomach and provide sleep

- Peppermint aids digestion lessens inflammation and muscle pain

- Jasmine empowers the immune system, curbs diabetes and lowers cholesterol

- Green tea is known as the healthiest drink after water in the world. It contains a great number of polyphenols that empowers heart and brain health. The small quantity of caffeine it contains helps to enhance fat burning.

- Black tea has enough compounds that help the heart, stress levels, and digestion.

Even though there are about 1-5 calories in a teacup, and it won't break you from the fasted state due to the small volume it contains.

Additionally, avoid brewing teas with fruit, berries or any other kinds of seasoning containing carbohydrates content. This is because the sugar in it will likely hold the beneficial advantages of autophagy.

Coffee. The simplest and best idea to suppress hunger during fasting is by drinking coffee because caffeine provides you with a jolt of energy and adds to your focus while enhancing fat burning.

Simultaneously, coffee possesses numerous health benefits like high polyphenol count, better blood sugar and lowered risk of Alzheimer's infection. So, it's a great booster for the mitochondria and brain.

To remain at a fasting state, continue to consume black coffee. Ordinarily adding a pinch of Stevia or Cinnamon, you could unknowingly end your fast. However, using a small quantity, like a few milligrams won't have any negative effect on your fasting. Also, instant coffee mixers possess some added ingredients that will end your fasted state.

Always be cautious of the amount of caffeine you drink.

Avoid consuming anything higher than 1-2 cups of coffee daily as it leads to caffeine intolerance and higher cortisol levels. Stress can stop you from ketosis but could as well prepare you to be more catabolic during fasting. Decaf, still, is potentially limitless, even though it contains caffeine also.

This makes me ask this question: Is it healthy to add butter to your coffee during fasting Bulletproof pattern?

Truly pure fat such as coconut oil, or MCT oil, butter, do not increase blood sugar; thus, it can put you in the semi-fasted mood. The fat won't go beyond the blood-brain barrier, and this will make your mind reason that it hasn't consumed anything.

However, this will hinder the process of autophagy even as the little amount of 50 calories keeps you into the fed mood and blocks the cell from self-digesting themselves.

Even though you'll lose some of the health benefits of detoxification, it's not an unhealthy thing, because it will equip you with energy and help you remain in ketosis.

From here, try to think of the reasons you're engaging in water fasting.

- If your reason for embarking on fasting is for weight loss and putting MCT oil or butter to your coffee is helpful to you then continue with it. Nevertheless, don't forget you'll need a small quantity intake of calories and adding all the sticks of butter into your cup will provide you with no less than one thousand calories.

- If your purpose is to clean your body against toxic proteins and inflammation carefully, then don't eat anything at all and engage in strict water fasting together with salt, mineral water, and teas.

Artificial Sweeteners. Is it possible to consume artificial sweeteners during water-fasting? Here lies the answer: It centers on the type of sweetener you're using, your reason for engaging in water fasting and how your system responds to them. So many sweeteners contain carbs in them, such as maltodextrin, dextrose or sucralose, try to avoid them.

Typical sweeteners such as Stevia doesn't have insulin or blood sugar, which makes them perfect for consumption.

Moreover, be cautious of how you specifically react to Stevia. Though it doesn't contain calories, it's 300 times sweeter than table sugar which could lead to placebo-like insulin response. That sweetness arouses your taste buds, which can make you end your fast - that's how powerful the mind is.

To make sure you don't fall into that trap, flee from all sweeteners during fasting, but if you can't, then test and experiment on them to see if it's suitable for your body.

Apple Cider Vinegar. Apple cider vinegar is a wonderful drink useful for fasting due to its anti-inflammatory and anti-bacterial compounds. It contains acidic substances but helpful in balancing your body's pH levels.

Apple cider vinegar has zero calories, and it possesses other minerals like potassium, iron and some amount of magnesium, suitable for fasting as it equips you to guide your electrolytes and curb deficiencies. Apple cider vinegar eliminates bad bacteria available in your gut and neutralizes hunger. Also, it can be joined with sparkling water to brew a fantastic tasty beverage.

Make sure to not take more than 1-2 tablespoons of ACV at a time to ensure you're not ending autophagy early.

Consuming it during your fasting period is okay and even better when breaking your fast. When breaking your fast put squeezed lemon juice to enhance the creation of digestive enzymes and ready your gut for eating. Try not to put lemon juice while fasting as it could pose the same placebo effect.

Mineral Water. Try to drink regular water, mineral, and sparkling water, because when you're engaging in fasting, you also flush out much water which may cause electrolyte imbalances and mineral deficiencies to your body. To avoid that, add a pinch of sea salt or pink Himalayan sea salt into your water. Additionally, when you consume ionized rock salt, it gives you iodine which encourages thyroid functioning and restricts hypothyroidism.

Help for Those New to Water Fasting

For decades, man has used this form of fasting for several reasons; however, this could be difficult at first for beginners, and that is the purpose of this section.

How to prepare for a fast

It is imperative to get your body prepped up for a fast before it commences. Intermittent fasting, as well as KD for a period of 2-3 weeks, is a good way to start. As your body gradually adapts to the new way of living, you can then extend the fasting period.

Just like a muscle, the more you train it, the bigger and stronger it becomes. So also, the more you fast, the easier it becomes. This is known as fasting fitness.

Another way to prep the body for what lies ahead is to go on a 20-24 hour fast weekly for a minimum of 1-2 weeks before commencing on the water fasting period. This strategy will help your body adapt to periods of abstinence from food:[27]

Cut down your schedule to have a low-stress level. Stress, especially at a high level, is one of the most discouraging factors while fasting. Therefore, it is expedient that you arrange your schedule in such a way that it becomes so light and you will still have time to rest and even take a vacation. This is very necessary especially at the early stages of water fasting when the body is just getting used to a new way of living. However, after developing a sufficient amount of fasting stamina, keep yourself engage to stay distracted especially when hunger sets in. Also, when the body is utilizing a large number of ketones, you are more active and productive.

If after trying so hard to adjust your schedule you still found out that you just can't escape from a high level of stress, then extended water fast is not ideal for you. You can try taking short and deep breaths once or twice daily.

Taking in short and deep breaths daily has a lot of health benefits. Short breaths boost the production of adrenaline as well as other fight and flight hormones which slows down the process of healing. Long and deep breath, however, produces the opposite effect by stimulating the healing process.

Try as much as possible to avoid negative people. There are two sets of people we are likely to come across in life:

- Positive people who encourage us to be the best that we can.

- Negative people who try as much as possible to drag you down.

You need to stay away from the second group of people during a fast as they could weaken your determination.

---

[27] Water Fasting: 12 Strategies to Prepare Properly - DrJockers.com. (2019). Retrieved from https://drjockers.com/water-fasting/

f such negative people are unavoidable (family member or workmates) why not sit hem down and have a heart-heart discussion with them. However, try not to act as a udge in the matter. Rather, explain your goals and the importance of the exercise to hem. You could be surprised at the effect of such conversation as they may suddenly become supportive.

Drink a lot of filtered water. Particularly if you are on an extended fast, hydration is vital. The reason is that your body depletes its sugar reservoir in the form of glycogen stored in the liver and muscles, so you lose water as well. Glycogen is lost alongside water, and once you deplete this source of energy, you will pass out the excess water. Also, the reduction in the levels of your insulin results in the excretion of additional sodium, and this would help your body to lose more water.

You would require access to enough clean water. It would be very helpful to get a very quality reverse osmosis system such as the Big Berkely water system or the iSpring that would make clean water easily available in your home. If this would not be possible, you can also buy bottled Fiji water from a nearby grocery store.

It is important to have a personal water system and drinking glasses or mason jars to lower the risk of plastic exposure. The Big Berkey and iSpring are inexpensive, and after a few months, the cost is lower, compared to buying the bottled Fiji water. Your goal should be to drink at least one ounce of water for every pound of your weight.

Get Some Quality Salts. While on an extended fast, electrolytes are required, and I recommend using high-quality salts like Himalayan Sea Salt, Celtic Sea Salt, and Redmond's Real Salt.

Like I earlier said, your insulin levels are reduced when you are fasting. Insulin is a hormone that functions in driving sugars into the body cells, and it also causes sodium retention. Reduced levels of insulin cause sodium to be excreted in high quantities.

When you start feeling light-headed or tired during the fast, place a pinch of salt on your tongue, then drink about 4 to 8 ounces of water. There is an instant increase in brain function and energy for most people.

Fix a spa day. Fasting helps you to save money since you won't be eating, I would advise that you rechannel that money to yourself. Schedule an appointment or two at the spa, enjoy the sauna, or get a message. All these can decrease stress, rid your body of toxins and make your fast less stressful.

As humans, we are naturally predisposed to gravitate towards pleasurable activities. One way we can do this is through food, and this is the reason a lot of us battle with food addictions. It is also the reason we usually feel a wide range of emotions while on a water fast. Our bodies have adapted to the neurochemical spike we get from food, so it would be difficult to adjust to the absence of this each day.

Fixing one or two spa days gives your body something positive to expect as a reward. You would be amazed at how this simple act can help you satisfy those emotions that you might experience in the course of the fast. The spa treatment causes you to expect something very nice as a form of personal reward.

If you can, avoid the kitchen. One of the major things most people have to battle against if they enter the kitchen is food cravings. I usually suggest that they try as much as possible to stay away from the kitchen. This is particularly important when you start fasting for the first time. After some time, you become mentally strong enough to avoid this temptation.

If it is impossible to stay away from the kitchen, get drinking water, or prepare herbal tea and make sure that you are drinking this while cooking in the kitchen. Drinking the water helps to suppress hunger and cravings for food.

Strategize your drinking times. Usually, you experience increased hunger at your usual feeding times. This is a natural and expected process that is caused by ghrelin, which is the hormone that is responsible for making you hungry. When you drink water, the level of ghrelin is lowered, resulting in lower levels of hunger as well. You can also consider drinking herbal teas like chamomile or green tea.

Take a fruity drink. If you are feeling very low during your course of water fasting, consider making a zero-calories lemonade by mixing liquid stevia and organic lemon juice to water. Drinking this mix would produce a boost in the neurotransmitters that would lift your mood; thus, making your water fast more fun.

Drinking a fruity drink is one of the things I enjoy doing most because it positively lifts my mood and makes the fast less uncomfortable and more enjoyable. My family and I enjoy the new natural water Stevia that is rich in fruit, and it is also excellent when added to water. You only need a little bit since it is very sweet and has zero calories or sugar.

Allow your feet to touch the ground every day. It can be particularly beneficial to make you put your bare feet on sand, grass or dirt. The Earth has some anions (negative ions) and rich electromagnetic frequency that can serve as antioxidants. We are unable to absorb anions due to the rubber soles on our shoes.

Walking in socks or barefoot on the Earth helps you to activate your body's electromagnetic current and feel enhanced energy, mental alertness, and relaxation. This is similar to having a bath and washing away all the Electromagnetic field that your body might have absorbed. Like a lot of us that like taking a bath or shower every day, it would be nice to cleanse your electromagnetic field every day by contact with the bare floor for 10 minutes or more.

It would be simpler to do this in warmer climates, compared to colder climates. Consider wearing socks or walking around your neighborhood when it is cold outside. Your neighbors might think you are a little odd, but the outcome would be pleasing. If you can afford to, you could also take a vacation to a hot, sunny beach for your fast when it is winter, and there are lots of snow.

If daily grounding isn't possible, don't worry, your fast would still be effective. Daily grounding would only make your fast less discomforting.

If you can, get sunshine every day. It is very helpful to get your body in the sun, although, make sure that you avoid getting a sunburn while catching that extra sunshine. A suntan enhances vitamin D and improves fat depletion that tilts your body system into ketosis.

Additionally, the sun has strong biophotons that can lower stress hormones and cause the production of excitatory neurotransmitters like dopamine, serotonin, and endorphins that would make you enjoy your fasting process more.

If you can afford to, this is an additional reason to take a vacation to the beach for your initial fast. Obviously, not all individuals can afford to do this, but you can still achieve excellent outcomes while fasting even in the absence of the sun, it only makes it even more enjoyable.

Set your body in motion. It can be extremely beneficial to go out and take walks all through the day. By nature, walking enhances the lymphatic and circulatory systems and increases excitatory neurotransmitters.

It is more advisable to take walks in a place filled with plants like the woods or a park so that you can get a contra-natural electromagnetic field from nature. If it is impossible or you are restricted by the weather, then take a walk in your home. You can also walk to and from the store, use a bike, treadmill or elliptical.

Your aim is not to use up your calories or work out. Walking is only a leisurely exercise to set your body in motion at a comfortable speed. The goal is to get a minimum of 40 to 60 minutes of leisurely movement every day divided into sections all through the day. You can divide it into 10 minutes- 4 to 6 times every day, 15 minutes- 3 to 4 times every day, or 20 minutes- 2 to 3 times every day. Select the method that would be suitable and convenient for you.

Fix relaxation periods. In the world today, we are constantly moving, and this makes us 'efficiency' addicts. Water fast enables you to live contrary to the way that we have become addicted to and allows you periods of rest, take a quick nap, have a warm bath, use some essential oils and to just enjoy yourself.

If you are water fasting for the first time, you might require additional rest compared to when you have been fasting intermittently for some time or if you have done at least one extended fast. With time, while you develop your fasting habit, and you notice that you are very efficient while water fasting, it might even be a better idea to engage yourself in pleasurable activities so that you would not have to think about food.

You are permitted to be busy when fasting only when you have adjusted, and you are beginning to enjoy it, but when you start feeling weak and tired, it is advisable to slow down and rest.

Chapter 6: Understanding your Fasting Routine

Finding the Most Suitable Eating Routine

If you are usually very busy, and you are always on the go, the most effective habit to adopt is one that you can adhere to and that you know you can accomplish. Even if there might be a daily variation in your fasting routine, it has to be effective enough for your lifestyle.

Consider how your days go and what would be most effective. For instance:

- 16-hour fasts on Monday, Wednesday and Friday

- 18-20 hour fasts on Tuesday, Thursday and Saturday, since you would be busier

Try not to worry excessively about your fasting and eating times. You might not feel like eating even when it is time to eat some times, if this happens, continue your fast.

One of the challenges of fasting that is hardly talked about is understanding how to handle yourself to the best of your capabilities. This is where the phrase, "different strokes for different folks" comes to play, so it is not realistic to recommend a particular method for everyone to use to enhance their energy and effectiveness. One thing that can be done by everyone to improve the efficacy and energy when on a fast is to manipulate your morning routine until you discover an effective method. This would be beneficial in getting the best out of your morning routine for optimum effectiveness and energy. There is no one-size-fits-all strategy. Discover the hours that are effective for your lifestyle and start with that.

As soon as you wake up, meditate for 15 minutes

Each morning, as soon as you get out of bed, place a pillow on the ground and sit on it, then engage in 15 minutes of meditation. It is quite hard to clear your mind while sitting since thinking of suppressing a thought is another form of thinking too. It might take time to be skilled at it, but as soon as you are, it can be very beneficial in ways like enhancing your capability to think, managing stress better, being more attentive and making rational decisions. Science has also proved that your brain can be improved physically through meditation. It does this by reducing the grey-matter in the amygdala, and this helps to reduce stress and worry, at the same time, the grey matter in the hippocampus- which is the area of memory and learning is increased.

Morning workouts: how to do it

If you prefer to work out in the morning, how do you handle working out while fasting? The problem with exercising in the morning is that you might lose muscle mass. The reason for this is that your body starts using up your muscle once protein is no longer available. Buying BCAAs is a waste of money because they do not help you gain or maintain your muscle and make sure to follow comfortable and light exercise routines. If you prefer workout after your workday, like in the evening, then working out while fasting shouldn't be a problem. It is an individual choice to eat before working out. Ensure that you still have carbs to energize you before exercising. If your dinner is two hours or more before exercising, eat protein together with carbs such as oats or sweet potato that takes a while to digest. If it would be less than two hours, you must eat a meal that digests easily. Fruits like banana or apple together with one protein scoop is an excellent idea. You should make your fasting routine to fit your lifestyle.

Establish a routine

Water Fasting entails going without food and taking only water for a certain period- from 12 hours to 40 days or more. To sustain their health, most people who fast regularly, fast for 24 hours once a week. Intermittent fasting is also practiced widely. There is a misconception that intermittent fasting causes weakness. This is untrue.

In contrast, it enhances your energy and health. After intermittent fasting, your energy level increases. At the beginning of your fast, your body stimulates the pituitary gland to secrete HGH (Human Growth Hormone). The increase in hormone makes your body to utilize additional fat as a fuel source, rather than degrading your muscle. There is no proof that a 72-hour fast would lower your muscle mass. If your weight reduces, it is as a result of fat reduction. A 24-hour fast is enough to sustain your health and energy. However, what happens in the case of a chronic health issue that requires a solution? Here, you would have to engage in long-term fasts that might range from 3 to 21 days, or even more. With the supervision of a professional, most illnesses can be cured by fasting moderately.

Planning the lengths of your fasts

Fix a timeframe for your water fast. Try starting with a 24-hour fast. If you are fasting alone, restrict your water fast to 3 days. There is some proof that fasting for a short period like 1-3 days is beneficial to health. If you would be fasting for a more extended period, ensure that it is under the guidance of a medical expert, like at a fasting retreat where a chiropractor or a medical expert can guide you. It might be less risky. Instead of long-term fasts for more than three days, periodic short-term fasts might be more beneficial. Try doing a water fast once a week.

Guidelines for fasting length and period

You can use Time Blocking to establish your routines. Time Blocking is when you fix a block of time for every meal period. I refer to this as 'directing your time.' Majority of the time, the instant we become adapted to fasting and no longer experience hunger pangs while fasting, eating becomes what we do only out of boredom. Or when we have a craving, or maybe time is moving too slow.

We tend to monitor the clock, asking ourselves: "How many hours left? Really, I can't eat for another 4 hours? How is that possible?" Time Blocking becomes essential here. This was the approach I frequently used in the early weeks of my fast, during the transitional phase of a ketogenic diet or intermittent fasting

These are a few tips for using Time Blocking when on a water fast

Plan your day one- or two-hour sections, make your primary task or activity for each time frame in a bullet format. You can do this with colorful highlighters or pens.

It is not necessary to be precise about what you have to do for each hour. It is acceptable to make non-specific statements about the things that you want to achieve.

Doctors recommend drinking extra water whether you are fasting or not so be mindful to include this. Include any multivitamins that might have been recommended by your doctor. Multivitamins and water would go a long way.

Make sure to include your fasting hour.

Ensure that your Block List is close to you at every time of the day and highlight or cancel out each block that represents a complete task. Since you now have a sense of direction, time would pass much faster, and you will be amazed by your effectiveness and cognizance

This is very effective for people who are homeschooled, corporate workers and homemakers, even those who have free work days. It is particularly beneficial to amateurs in water fasting and for a lengthier fasting period.

Longer is greater: advantages of Fasting for up to 3 days

When fasting, longer is better, although your goals will determine how long you fast. It is not better generally, but for longevity, protection against cancer, stronger immunity and anti-aging, it can be a good option. Walter Longo, a prolific USC researcher, has carried out extensive research on the 'stronger immunity' benefit.

In Longo and his colleague's research published in Cell,[28] they explained the primary metabolic events after long periods of 3-day fasts. Participants produced additional white blood cells- that implies improved immunity, after 3 days. The benefit of protection against cancer was discovered too. Longo discovered that both cancer patients who were undergoing therapy and healthy people benefited health-wise, after fasting for 3 days. Like other cells in the body, cancer cells get nourishment from glucose, fasting deprives cancer cells of glucose, resulting in their deaths and this can help to protect against cancer later.

Limiting calorie intake every day helps to rid the body of the by-products of cells, fasting for 3-5 days uses up the entire glycogen in the body, thereby clearing even more by-product from the cells.

Strategies for Extended Fasting

There are unlimited methods to reap the benefits of fasting, and I will be discussing some of this that pertains to extended fasting:

- Modern- this strategy infuses caffeine in addition to some multivitamins

- Minimalist- this strategy involves salts- as a source of electrolytes and water

They are both beneficial, but this is determined by how determined you are to follow the rules of extended fasting.

---

[28] Cheng, C., Adams, G., Perin, L., Wei, M., Zhou, X., & Lam, B. et al. (2014). Prolonged Fasting Reduces IGF-1/PKA to Promote Hematopoietic-Stem-Cell-Based Regeneration and Reverse Immunosuppression. *Cell Stem Cell*, *14*(6), 810-823. doi: 10.1016/j.stem.2014.04.014

Minimalist Strategy. As the name suggests, the minimalist fasting strategy is minimal. It simulates a primitive period perfectly. There was no caffeine for our forefathers to use to suppress hunger, and neither was there BCAA (Branched Chain Amino Acid) to prevent loss of muscle. Although a few advocates of fasting suggest that caffeine does not stop the fast, one cup of coffee will inhibit some fasting processes. Also, BCAAs generate a response to insulin, which would inhibit some other fasting processes. This strategy involves going without foods, exclusively drinking water (while including a pinch of salt), and no multivitamins at all

Modern Strategy. This strategy infuses some modern inventions while producing the benefits of long-term fasting. It involves tea and coffee, which have the least possible calories and also represses hunger. This makes fasting easier for people who might feel intense hunger pangs.

A few people use supplements like BCAAs and exogenous ketones. Exogenous ketones stimulate the process of utilizing ketones (gotten from fat) as a fuel source and BCAAs prevent muscle loss.

Make sure to select the exogenous ketone carefully that you would be using; the most popular ketone is BHB (Beta-hydroxybutyrate) which contains MCT powder that is enriched with calories and can bring you out of your fast.

Suggested Timetable for Water Fasts

- Stage 0- One week of a reduced normal diet

- Stage 1- At least two weeks of low-fat cleansing diet

- Stage 3- Drink water exclusively for 3-5 days.

- Stage 4- 1-4 days of steamed vegetables, miso soup, and fresh fruit juice.

- Stage 5- 5-14 days of a low-fat cleansing diet

Timetable for 3-day Fast

A 3-day fast might appear more challenging than it really is. The hardest part of a 3-day fast is stopping the fast at the end (we will discuss this later)

This timetable was constructed based on Tim Ferriss' experience. Going on 70% of the fast during the weekend may prevent disruptions in your work days during the week.

- 8pm, Thursday- Round up your last meal and start your fast.

- 8am, Friday- For 3-4 hours, start walking. Doing this uses up your glycogen reserves and helps to change your energy source for glucose to fat. If you prefer to drink coffee first, do so, it might be helpful. While walking, you could listen to audiobooks or make a call

- Friday/Saturday - If you are free to go on extended walks at any time, go. Total depletion of glycogen reserves takes 28-48 hours, though this is determined by your experience and diet. The process is faster when you walk for more extended periods.

NOTE: Ensure that you are drinking enough water, but not excessively. Drink water only when you are thirsty. Drinking too much water might wash away a lot of electrolytes from your body. To prevent this too, include a pinch of salt. The most difficult part of going on a 3-day fast is not the hunger pangs but ending the fast.

Return to Normal: Regular Diet

Individual requirements, emotional, physical and spiritual state determines the period that would be spent on these stages to prepare and recover from water fasting.

NOTE: One day of water fasting is equal to one day of recovery, if you engage in water fasting for ten days, then you should rest for a minimum of 10 days before any intense activity.

End of the Day routine and meditation (coupled with meditation techniques)

Yoga, together with meditation at the end of the day will improve your mood. A few of the best yoga practices can happen when you have no food in your system. You might even sense your internal organs as you dig deeper and tap into the meditation during yoga while you are fasting. You don't have to feel like your energy is insufficient for yoga, it is good to do something mild, but if you regularly practice yoga, it feels nice to twist the spaces that do not exist on a normal day in your body. While on a fast, meditation can be more intense. It is exciting to sense your mind becoming peaceful very fast, like turning in a switch. If you are regularly eating, it might take a minimum of half the time spent during a one-hour meditation to experience the peace; whereas, if you are fasting, it is easier to experience the peace while meditating, and achieve the feeling of 'nothing' that experienced yogis reach with equal experience and silence

You can engage in the following activities:

- Spine Healing Session.

- Yoga Nidra Session

- Sound Healing Therapy

- Transformational Breathing Therapy

- Thai Box and Chi

- Mandala Painting Session

When your internal organs are left to rest, without expending energy on digestion, there is a more intense cleansing that leads to cell renewal. It is similar to pressing a reset button internally. There is improved absorption of vitamins and minerals that reduce the space that food can be absorbed while getting an equal feeling of satiety and health benefits. This period is also beneficial for tissues and glands producing smooth skin and clearer eyes.

Chapter 7: Ending the Water Fasting Process the Proper Way

Since you won't be consuming solid food while embarking on a water fast, your digestion might not be able to handle your regular diet at the beginning. When you eat too many hard-to-digest foods after breaking your water fast, it could lead to devastating outcomes.

Below is a list of foods you can follow to easily and properly break a water fast and shun any potential complications within the process.

- Fruit juice

- Vegetable juice

- Raw fruit and green leafy vegetables

- Yogurt

- Vegetable soup and cooked vegetables

- Cooked grains and beans

- Milk, dairy, and eggs

- Meat, fish, and poultry

Everything Else

The listed foods are orderly arranged on how challenging they will be to digest. At the top of the list are the easily digestible ones, while the difficult-to-digest ones are listed at the bottom.

After breaking your water fast, endeavor to start with the foods at the top of the list and gradually move down to the hard ones. You can add more foods from the list, with every meal.

For example: End the water fast using orange juice, which is found in group list #1, later on, eat a banana which is #3. When you find out that your system is okay, prepare a small amount of salad and top it with yogurt, as you can see in food groups #4 and #5 as the next food in line.

Endeavor to break your fast with a small number of meals making sure to leave two hours of space apart. After adding food continuously to the list, you can begin increasing the number of your meals.

If your fasting lasted for two days, it's possible you won't have any issues when you end your fast, and there shouldn't be any issues with going back to your old diet right from the beginning. However, if your fasting lasted for a week or more, then it will take time to transition back into your normal diet pattern gradually.

The overall rule is, the more hours you fasted, the wiser and more cautious you should be when ending the fast. Irrespective of how little the time you take to fast is, there won't be any problem if you take time to get back to your normal diet easily.

However, depending on the hours you fasted, it could take you from 1-4 days before your digestion can be 100% in order again.

The simple truth is, not everybody will follow the laid down guide provided, it's fine to skip one or two during the process, but it's healthier to keep it in mind as a general guide.

Things to Avoid Drinking and Eating When Ending Your Fast

Stay away from fried foods or anything with much oil, or even added fats as they're difficult to digest.

Avoid all high-carbohydrate foods; like pizza, pasta, white rice, and bread. Carbohydrate foods not only have zero calories, but they also affect blood sugar levels. A quick change in blood sugar levels will affect the smoothness of your fasting and will harm the benefits attached to fasting, like fat loss and added insulin sensitivity.

Avoid anything containing refined or processed sugars; content such as high fructose corn syrup, table sugar, and agave nectar. The way you're trying to shun filling your caloric limits during your fasting periods with empty calories, ensure you don't rubbish those 500 or 600 calories on simple sugars.

In fulfilling your sweet tooth, try honey and maple syrup which are two sweeteners that are good choices when consumed at moderation. Also, processed sugars are to be avoided in those two days a week you'll engage in fasting. If staying away from sugar is difficult, try remembering that it's only twice a week you'll be going without it.

Furthermore, avoiding sugar intake twice-a-week will help you combat sugar addiction.

Add sweetener and other additives to your coffee with caution. Although only one cup of black coffee contains five insignificant calories, 260 calories can be gained from drinking one 16oz. Mocha- if the whipped cream is included, that cup of coffee becomes 330 calories.

Avoid sports drinks, regular soda, juices, or diet soda. It is usual for most Americans to get about 140-180 calories every day from sweet beverages such as sports drink and soda. Stay away from the diet forms too.

Alcohol. In a 2012 research, it was discovered that Americans drink alcoholic beverages that contain about 300 calories each day. This might appear insignificant but think about the accumulated value gotten in one week. However, a lot of people even drink more than that every day.

One hundred twenty-five calories are contained in one 5-oz glass of red wine. One standard 12-oz beer has caloric content higher than 125, and diet cola and double vodka contains an alarming 258 calories. Indulging in any of these drinks can increase your caloric restrictions on the days when you are fasting.

Unhealthy foods such as pretzels, chips, buttery popcorn, candy, fruit snacks, etc. One of the numerous advantages of fasting is the purification of the body. Eating unhealthy foods which are notably filled with ingredients that are deficient in some nutrients while fasting will, in reality, produce more poisons in addition to the ones your body is trying to eliminate. Rather than eating these unhealthy foods, eat only natural, whole or unpackaged foods when you are fasting as well as ending a fast.

Eating After a Water Fast

A few people engage in this type of fasting to improve their health- weight loss or toxin elimination. Others use water fasting to get a clear head and enter into the state of meditation. Regardless of the purpose of the fast, the fast would come to an end, and you will have to start eating. It doesn't matter if your fast is only short-term, be careful of when you begin eating again.

Step 1: On the morning of the day after your fast ended, mix one part water with one part fruit or vegetable and drink. If you can, use a juicer to produce your juice. The less concentrated juice would provide nourishment without causing a disturbance in your digestive system.

Step 2: On the afternoon of the day after your fast ended, drink one cup of chicken broth or vegetable. If you like, eat plain crackers or a piece of bread together with the broth. Keep drinking the juice mix. The soup provides additional nourishment and primes your digestive system for normal foods.

Step 3: On the evening of the day after your fast ended, drink a more substantial soup like minestrone or vegetables. Eat a bit of undressed salad together with vegetables and fresh fruits. Consume one glass of juice that is not diluted with water.

Step 4: On the second day after your fast ended, keep eating the vegetables and fresh fruits, juices, and fruits. In the evening, you can include dairy products like yogurt or milk.

Step 5: On the fourth day, continue with your regular feeding routine. Beginning from the third or fourth day, start including other whole foods that are cooked like meat, fish, nuts, eggs, whole grains and uncooked fruits and vegetables. Ensure that your legumes and grains are cooked thoroughly since this is to soften them and make them easily digestible. On the fifth day, you are free to include non-cultured dairy products like milk, and meat or eggs. Ensure that your meals contain low-fat so that you do not overwhelm your digestive system. Though it is usually recommended, cooked vegetables, fresh juices, and organic fruits are unnecessary.

How Long the Gradual Process Should Take to Get Back to "Normal"

Due to the dormancy of your digestive system, the transit from a fast is very significant. Your system is still unable to digest, but you have to gradually revive it, reverently, by consuming foods that are easy to digest in tiny portions. If not, it would be very uncomfortable. The same way the remnant of food in the gut at the start of long-term fast decay, it can happen in this case too. Except for basic fruits and vegetables, or juices, any other food remains in the stomach, till your digestive system is capable of digesting. This process may take days to finish. After a fast, the period of restoration of healthy feeding with a regular appetite is as long as the duration of the actual fast.

When ending a water fast, constipation might result in the first few days. Constipation happens due to the sharp increase in fiber and food consumption. To lower the risks of constipation, drink adequate fluids around 6-8 oz. Glasses of fluid every day all through the day and slowly increase food consumption. Make sure to avoid going back to your previous fasting habits. Fasting would be less beneficial for your health if you go back to consuming meals rich in fat and sugar later. The health advantages of your fast can be maintained by eating a low-sodium diet that is high in whole grains, fruits or vegetables, or a diet low in fat.

Engage in 30 minutes of a workout five days a week. Adopt a healthy lifestyle to enhance your health and general wellness, allocate only a small portion to fasting.

Chapter 8: Tips and Tricks Water Fasting Success

Relationship Between Autophagy and Ketogenic Diet

Some things are dependent on one another such as water fasting, the ketogenic lifestyle, and autophagy. One of the more popular methods of activating autophagy is by undergoing a ketogenic diet.

Before proceeding, it is essential to note that the Ketogenic Diet does not enhance your capability to go without eating- every machine requires an energy source. The mechanism by which keto works is by providing your body with a method of using a more persistent energy source obtained from heavy fats instead of carbohydrates. Normally, people who are not used to the Ketogenic Diet experience hunger pangs when they do not eat snacks for a few hours. These hanger pangs can be regularly seen in people that are dependent on quickly depleted carbs. If you already have previously adapted to keto, you should be able to function without food for days and without any need to eat.

Fasting lowers the level of insulin and blood sugar which promotes the secretion of hormones that deplete fats, like adrenaline and glucagon. This then supports the degradation of fats known as triglyceride reserves in adipose tissue. Eventually, when triglycerides are transported to the liver, they are used as a source of fuel or to generate ketone bodies. Once your ketone levels become about 7-8 mmol/L that's when you know your body has begun ketosis.[29]

As a result of reduced carbohydrate intake, the ketogenic diet results in a decrease in the levels of insulin and glucose. Contrary to fasting, some amount of protein and foods rich in fats are permitted. Unlike glucose, fats and proteins do not significantly affect the levels of blood glucose.

Contrarily, fat does not have this effect, eating a diet rich in fat, but low in protein and carbs divert your energy source to ketone bodies and imitates a natural, fasted condition. This means that by being in a ketotic state, you would be stimulating autophagy.[30]

[29] Paoli, A. (2014). Ketogenic Diet for Obesity: Friend or Foe?. *International Journal Of Environmental Research And Public Health*, *11*(2), 2092-2107. doi: 10.3390/ijerph110202092

[30] Takagi, A., Kume, S., Maegawa, H., & Uzu, T. (2016). Emerging role of mammalian autophagy in ketogenesis to overcome starvation. *Autophagy*, *12*(4), 709-710. doi: 10.1080/15548627.2016.1151597

Furthermore, lowering your intake of protein and carbohydrates, in turn, lowers the number of poisonous substances that are absorbed by your body, so there is just a little toxin for your body to eliminate, making autophagy even more fully effective.

This is probably why people that engage in the keto diet start feeling like an improved version of themselves. Their bodies are eliminating toxins, and there is an upgrade in their health.

One of the main proponents of the ketogenic diet is water fasting because digesting even the healthiest meals uses energy and can stress the body eventually. Water fasting helps the body to rest and permits recycling of excess energy.

Additionally, the body enters into a ketotic state more rapidly if you are on a water fast. Water fasting creates extended, more efficient periods of ketosis. Also, a more intense restoration at cellular levels is observed while on a water fast.

Even though this is similar to what happens on a Ketogenic Diet, but water fasting makes the process faster with the additional advantages we have discussed previously.

The type of fat used to generate ketones is one other difference between water fasting and a keto diet. Fat reservoirs are the source of fat when you are on a fast. However, the fat in keto is gotten from the high-fat meals you are consuming. The quantity of calories gotten from your dietary fat determines if a ketogenic diet would result in weight loss.

Start Fasting Gradually

It might be challenging to undergo a water fast, but your body starts to adapt to the recent changes eventually. Within the first three days, you might be tempted to stop. The smell of food excites you, and you will start to imagine all the foods you would get to eat after breaking your fast. By day three, ketosis is complete, and you will start to feel dizzy if you get up too fast, have intense headaches, and sleep disturbances.

After two weeks, you would no longer feel the intense headaches and hunger pangs. You might still feel dizzy and very cold because the levels of your blood pressure are still lower than normal. By then you can easily cook family meals without temptations, and you would begin to detest the smell of sugary snacks and unhealthy foods.

In comparison to the first two weeks, the third week should be easier because this is because the body is adapting to the recent changes and you have eliminated the majority of the toxins in your body lowering flu-like and discomforting after effects.

Begin with a small fast. How many hours can you go without food? Three hours? Six hours? Begin with that and gradually add one hour every day.

Remember: Before you start running – learn to walk first.

Most people make the common error of starting directly with 24-hour fasts when they are used to 3-6 meals each day together with snacks. In some cases, it is possible to attempt this, but it might begin to feel like torture and starvation.

Eating the Right Foods

On fasting days, eat a little bit of food. Generally, fasting entails partially or completely going without food or drinks for a certain period.

Though it is possible to exclude food completely on fasting days, a few fasting strategies such as the 5:2 diet permits you to eat about 25% of your calorie needs in one day.[31]

If you are thinking of starting a fast, limit your caloric intake to enable yourself to eat small quantities during your fasting days. Limiting your intake can be healthier than engaging in a complete fast when you're starting as a beginner.

This method might help to lower the risks of fasting like experiencing hunger, inability to concentrate or light-headedness.

Because you do not feel really hungry, it might also make it easier to continue with the fast.[32]

Ensure Adequate Hydration. It is important to drink sufficient amounts of liquid while on a fast because thirst, fatigue, headaches, and dry mouths can be caused by mild dehydration.

Many health experts advise people to use the 8 by 8 rule- 8 glasses that are 8 oz. in size (less than 2 liters) of liquid each day- to ensure adequate hydration.

Although this might be enough, the quantity of liquid you need depends on you as an individual. It is very easy to become dehydrated while fasting because 20-30% of the

[31] Varady, K., Bhutani, S., Church, E., & Klempel, M. (2009). Short-term modified alternate-day fasting: a novel dietary strategy for weight loss and cardioprotection in obese adults. *The American Journal Of Clinical Nutrition*, *90*(5), 1138-1143. doi: 10.3945/ajcn.2009.28380

[32] Heilbronn, L., Smith, S., Martin, C., Anton, S., & Ravussin, E. (2005). Alternate-day fasting in nonobese subjects: effects on body weight, body composition, and energy metabolism. The American Journal Of Clinical Nutrition, 81(1), 69-73. doi: 10.1093/ajcn/81.1.69

fluid required by your body comes from food.

While fasting, a lot of people try to drink 2-3 liters (8.5-13 cups) of water throughout the day. But, thirst should guide you on when it is time to drink additional water, follow the instructions that your body is telling. Only you know when too much water is too much.

Eat Plenty of Protein. For most people, fasting is a form of weight loss although you have to remember that a reduction in caloric intake will make you lose not just fat but muscle as well.

One method of reducing the risk of losing muscle while on a fast is to make sure that you are consuming sufficient amount of proteins on the days that you are allowed to eat food.[33]

Also, adding protein to the small-sized meals on your fast days can help suppress your hunger and provide other beneficial effects.

Some researchers propose that getting 30% of your calories by eating protein can significantly suppress your appetite.[34]

Because of this, some bad after effects of fasting can be reduced by consuming some form of good protein.

Avoid ending your Fasts With large Meals. After fasting for a while, the thought of ending your fast with a large meal can be enticing but ending you fast with a large meal can make you weak and bloated. Also, if you desire to lose weight, large meals might impede your fasting objectives by impeding or stopping your weight loss process.

Eating too many calories after a fast lowers your caloric deficit because your total caloric intake affects your health, so the most effective way of ending a fast is to keep eating normally and continue with your usual eating schedule

Exercise while fasting. Before starting any workout routine, consult your doctor, especially when you are fasting. Your doctor knows your medical history and can specifically advise you on what to do. Also, tell your doctor about your wish to fast and your workout routine, so your doctor would know if this is suitable or unsafe.

Stop the fast and workout if you experience any discomfort or pain when exercising, or the aftereffects of a fast, and you are advised to call your doctor instantly. Your doctor would decide if your heart can cope with exercises when you are on a fast.

---

[33] Cava, E., Yeat, N., & Mittendorfer, B. (2017). Preserving Healthy Muscle during Weight Loss. *Advances In Nutrition: An International Review Journal, 8*(3), 511-519. doi: 10.3945/an.116.014506

[34] Leidy, H., Mattes, R., & Campbell, W. (2007). Effects of Acute and Chronic Protein Intake on Metabolism, Appetite, and Ghrelin During Weight Loss*. *Obesity, 15*(5), 1215-1225. doi: 10.1038/oby.2007.143

How does it feel to workout while fasting? This is determined by many factors, ranging from the fasting approach you use to the response of your body has to the fast. Following your body's directions is pertinent. If fasting makes you too tired to exercise, solve your nutrition issues first, then you can exercise later.

Although safety should be your priority, a number of exercise routines can enhance fasting.

Schedule your meals around your exercises. Cardio can be done on an empty stomach. You are allowed to go on a jog or register for that early morning spin session. However, it is vital to select the right foods before you attempt any form of cardio.

Since you know you would be working out, you should carefully select what to eat on the previous day as determined by how hard you would be exercising. For instance, you may want to increase your glycogen reserves by eating complex carbohydrates for dinner, the previous night so that you would be provided with easily accessible energy for your cardio exercise. It is inadvisable to do cardio when your stomach is full because the muscle's abrupt demand for blood diverts the important blood required for nutrient digestion and absorption. The best thing is to make plans beforehand to ensure that your nutrition provides the nutrients for your intense exercise, even though you would be exercising the following morning.

Exercise Suggestions For You

Choose less stressful exercises. While on a fast, a simple exercise might be very helpful because it makes sure that your body does not convert protein to an energy source.

While fasting, your body is dependent on energy reserved in the form of glycogen (this is the form in which glucose is stored by your body) If it has been a while since you last ate, your glycogen reserved might have been depleted, this would drive your body to use protein as a source of energy.

- Rather than working out by running, walk. Moderate walks are a less stressful way of increasing your heart rate.

- Engage in Tai Chi or light yoga. Gradual, precise movements stabilize and enhance your body, and this old approach is a popular way of clearing and soothing the mind.

- Engage in light yard chores or gardening. Gardening needs you to lift, bend or move in other ways. Yard work and gardening are both excellent activities that mimic exercise.

However the intense exercise may be, the moment you start to feel dizzy or weak, stop the exercise instantly. You might have to drink water and eat a small portion of food to bring your energy level back up.

The great thing is that engaging in less stressful workouts while fasting makes the body to start using fat as a source of energy. For people that are trying to lose weight, this is very beneficial.

Make sure your workout routine is practical. Rather than walking, you might feel like running, or you might feel that you can cope with lifting heavy weights. However, fasting alters the normal limits of your body.

If your fast is for a religious purpose, or a medical reason, make plans to include less stressful workouts that you can easily do. You can continue with your regular workout routine as soon as your fast has ended.

If your fast extends from dusk to dawn, you have to stay away from working out during those periods and make sure to workout at a time that is close to your eating periods in the morning or evening.

If the purpose of your fast is to lose weight or other health reasons, you have to include exercises with caution. Take care to do less stressful workouts on your fasting days, and engage in rigorous exercises on days that you eat extra calories.

When to Stop Working Out During Fasting. When fasting or working out, the most important thing to do is what your body is telling you because there is a large risk of reduction in the levels of your blood glucose. So if you have never done this before, do not register for a rigorous session that might involve maximum exertion of your heart. Do not overdo it. Overdoing it might make you feel light-headed or even lose consciousness due to a quick reduction in the levels of your blood glucose, and it is a scary situation when that happens.

A little bit of planning would be very beneficial. The most vital factor to consider while on an extended or intermittent fast is what your breakfast looks like and how it works well with your workout routine. It is vital to consume healthy fats, protein, organic fibers, and complex carbs during the eating period to sustain a healthy fast.

So, that's it. Rigorous, or less rigorous exercises, make sure to make suitable plans for your meals. Remember, the most important thing is to listen to your body. Do not engage in rigorous workouts if it's telling you not to do them. Throughout the fast, there will be a variation in your energy levels, from experiencing weakness and tiredness to experiencing energy bursts. Regardless of how energetic you feel, do not stress yourself. Rather, engage in calm, soothing yoga. Yoga is a gentle way of stretching out your muscles and engaging in mild exercises.

For some people, light stretches and yoga might be easy, and for others, it might be too rigorous. Do what makes you feel good and go from there.

The Significance of Sleep While Fasting

During water fasting, sleep is the next crucial thing after water intake. While sleeping, the body undergoes repair, restoration, detoxification, and metabolism. It also begins a growth phase where it stores up energy and the cells begin to grow. You're at an optimal state after a satisfactory 7-8 hours of sleep during fasting, and the rate of tissue renewal is increased while sleeping as opposed to being in an active state. Both sleep and fasting should complement each other to attain a better healthy body overall; therefore, a great advantage of fasting is its positive effect on sleep. Although during the fast, you may find it difficult to sleep as a result of the earlier energy surge, there will be a significant positive change in the pattern of sleep because of the regulation carried out by the body to bring back normalcy.

Professional Guidance During Water-Fasting

With proper medical supervision and adequate guidance, water fasting is an efficient and harmless way of assisting the body in self-restoration. However, like any other things that affect the body, there are some associated risks. For anyone that is considering undergoing a therapeutic fast, my advice would be to do this under the guidance of a certified IAHP expert who is trained in the process. The International Association of Hygienic Physicians consists of primary care doctors that are experts at supervising therapeutic fasts. Every approved member is a licensed osteopath, medical doctor or chiropractor, that has finalized at least a 6-month residency program at an authorized institution that is specialized in therapeutic fasts. Unlike in the past, fasting is now easily accessible due to the increase in the number of licensed professionals

Advantages of fasting under professional guidance. Maximum health is sustained when the body has adequate health requirements such as proper environment, psychology, and diet. If any of these requirements are inadequate, it affects your health. Most times, therapeutic fasting is an incredibly effective way of health recovery since it enables the body to produce an exceptional response to healing.

No other form of fasting can mimic the benefits of this way of fasting. Fasting, in a busy, noisy, or unsupportive surrounding will deprive the body of the chance to optimize the processes of self-restoration. Total rest is pertinent to optimize the beneficial effects of therapeutic fasting. Drinking juices exclusively or eating particular foods are essential as well. There are tremendous benefits both health and physiologically-wise when you consume these foods. However, this does not imply that the elimination diet, otherwise known as juice diet, is better than a straight water fast.

How A Chiropractor Will Help With The Fasting Process

Certain specialists in the health care sector concentrate on recognizing, and treating diseases that affect the junction between muscles and nerves, and they are very particular about curing these diseases by molding and sometimes, even altering the spinal cord. These specialists are called Chiropractors.

Chiropractors educate their patients on how to care for themselves by ergonomics, exercising, making user-friendly systems and other remedies to relieve back pain. Their main aim is to lessen the pain felt by patients and to increase their performance.

They believe that periodic fasting purges the body of harmful substances and causes the body to perform optimally.

There are certain criteria chiropractors take heed of during a fast;

First on the list of criteria is preventing death. Chiropractors expect side effects of fasting such as irritability, skin rashes, foul taste in the mouth, headaches, nausea and vomiting, unusual discharges from mucous membranes, postural hypertension and low back pain in the initial stage of fasting as a result of referral activity from kidney changes.

These professionals know that their patients undergo characteristic restorative crisis whereby persistent illnesses develop into short term illnesses and that it can be very distressing. Thus, their responsibility is to detect the boy's attempt to recover through a short term illness.

They are very mindful of carrying out the proper clinical supervision of their patients, after which they monitor the reaction of the body to the fast to determine the extent and severity of the therapy. To a great length, chiropractors monitor patient's activities like the food they eat, the time they sleep, and even as far as how susceptible they are to levels of stress.

Chiropractors can guarantee a risk-free experience, influencing the slightest reaction to water fasting (including hydration), as a result of the control they have over the patient's activities.

Chapter 9: How to Deal with Hunger During Water Fasting

It's crucial to note that starving yourself for fasting won't lead to death. This is pessimistic thoughts with fear works like a prophecy.

When you are a couple of minutes into a fast, and feeling hungry, telling yourself you can't do it, and the next meal you're going to eat dominates your mind, it's not going to take you anywhere.

Your body as a human has been transformed to control periods of fasting. Even when you come to think of it, there's no evolutionary logic attached to eating 3-5 meals per day. Naturally, we don't have anything like 3-5 sure meals on a daily. Too much availability of food only became possible in this new era.

Understand the Difference Between Psychological and Physical Hunger

Circadian clocks afford animals to predict daily events instead of ordinarily reacting to them. Also, the cells that create ghrelin possess circadian clocks that probably synchronize the expectation of food with metabolic cycles. In a nutshell, this means that eating a set of meals per day is trained and mastered behavior.

Most times we seem that we are hungry, we're not feeling true physiological or body hunger, rather what we're experiencing is psychological or head hunger. Immediately we notice this, then all it will take is to be disconnected from it until our system adapts to the fasting routine.

My Experience

In theory, fasting seems very easy. You could be thinking - yeah I will only avoid eating for some days and then continue with your meal afterward, but it goes beyond that. Personally, I have taken part in every type of fasting and failed several times. Every attempt I make looks pretty simple at the beginning. I used to be very excited concerning my latest plan that even the thought of eating never comes to my mind, I'd be so confident that I could bet on my success.

I'm committed at the starting of every fast, that I would choose to stick with one Meaning it's not until 20hrs plus that the interest of the fast starts to depreciate, and begin to lose the motivating spirit to keep going. However, now I understand that wha kept me quitting was that I thought I would reach the initial slump, which is unavoidable because everyone fasting goes through it as well. To me seems as if my brain is testing me to know if this is really what I desire.

It will be obvious to you when you hit the slumping state because, at that point, you'll be asking yourself whether you're doing the right thing, the mind will randomly remind you to eat something. But if you can be able to defeat that urge, you'll be empowered to continue your fast. That slump should be seen as a battle, in which you must fight and win to accomplish your goal. Make sure you're prepared for it and also expect it.

Fasting isn't an easy task, The beginning might be interesting to you, but it becomes tougher as time progresses, to the extent that you'll feel like giving up and eating anything in the cupboard or even buying a pizza to sustain the moment. AVOID DOING IT.

Follow this advice to succeed. Do yourself a favor and be sure to practice these tips before giving up.

- Always expect hunger

- Draft a plan detailing your strategy when you begin to feel the hunger

Take Tea or Coffee Without Adding Sugar

Everyone knows that caffeine provides you with energy, but not everyone knows it's a potent appetite suppressant. Coffee/tea can be used to stop the urge to eat for the whole day. Drinking hot tea or coffee can help in making a person feel as if he or she has eaten. Also, the truth that you're drinking something tasty makes it feel a lot like a meal.

Here's the question, should you use milk or not?

When your aim of fasting is to shed weight, then adding a small quantity of milk to your drink is healthy while those who are fasting for religious reasons or cleansing could brew their drink without adding milk.

If you prefer to be very strict, consume it black, although it doesn't make so much difference. You could add a dash of milk (not more than 6ml) and still be in a fasted state.

- Caffeine in tea/coffee represses your appetite

- Adding milk won't stop your fast

Ensure You're Drinking Plenty of Water

Thirst can appear like hunger. It might seem as if you're starving, but in the real sense, you're dehydrating. During fasting, a lot of water is removed from your body. Consume 2-3 liters of water daily when fasting. Lethargy and headaches are notable signs of dehydration, so when you experience these during fasting, drink more and more water. But if you aren't feeling the thirst to drink enough water, it could be that you've gotten to balance of salt-to-water in your blood. To solve this problem, add a small pinch of pink Himalayan salt into your water. It will also contribute to your electrolytes too.

Water is wonderful as it makes you feel fulfilled, but don't over consume it. Drinking massive amounts of water frequently will do more harm to you than good. The idea is to drink water whenever you feel hungry because consuming water unnecessarily will only make you urinate frequently and this flushes out your electrolytes that may cause flu-like symptoms. Make sure to stick with 2-3 liters and space out your durational consumption, and you'll be okay.

- Drink it when hunger comes knocking

- 2-3 liters every day

- Spread the water intake throughout the entire day

Go to Bed

It's baffling to note that a lot of people don't know that sleeping equals fasting as well.

The evening is the peak time that most people will break their fast, including me. I'll abide by it every day, then when evening comes around, I give in and join my family during dinner. Whenever this happens, I see it as a failure in my part by writing off the week and starting anew on Monday of another week. The whole thing will want to repeat itself over and over again.

I have realized going to bed earlier would help me succeed that hard part, and waking up 8 hrs later it would've been the next morning. It's very hard to break your fast in the night if you follow this trick. Breaking your fast will make you feel bad the next day, rather than good, so try to sleep and see whether you'll still be hungry by morning.

It's advisable to begin your fast before going to bed, and using this strategy will make your first 8 hrs of fasting much easier and hunger-free.

- If you desire to give up when evening comes around, fight that urge off strongly

- Try to sleep whenever you're hungry at night

Remember that hunger comes in waves. It will pass.

Many people don't understand how long hunger takes because they're prompted to eat something whenever they get little feeling of hunger. They're always afraid of the word "hunger" and began to eat anytime their system churns with hunger. Those who are used to fasting know that if you endure a bit, the hunger will leave. Just put it in your mind you'll eat later because even feelings of hunger don't take more than 20 minutes or so, which starts to reduce as time passes.

Hunger is as a result of increased ghrelin. That is, ghrelin increases when you begin fasting, which leads to hunger. The increased levels of ghrelin don't remain permanent, meaning hunger reduces as fasting continues. During your weight loss journey ensure you also have this in mind. When the hiccups come around during that feeling of hunger remember to tell yourself: "This feeling of hunger in me will vanish soon" then move on with your fasting.

- Hunger pangs only stay for 20 minutes before it starts to vanish

- Your hormone ghrelin causes the feeling of hunger

- The level of ghrelin reduces during ketosis

Distract Yourself

Human beings tend to mistake boredom for hunger. We tend to eat whenever we're bored because it keeps us busy. I was ignorant of how much eating food took out of my time during the day until I began to fast. I use to think that only the time spent on a meal is only the time we took to eat, but it was wrong. Thinking of what to consume at breakfast, lunch, dinner and what we'll eat during those times takes out a considerable amount of time spent because we spend much time thinking about it before eventually eating it.

It doesn't make sense when we start fasting, and our mind is still preoccupied with food. This happens because we have our normal day wired out of habit to be around food. So much so that even when you're not hungry, your system still triggers you to consume something as you keep thinking about it throughout the day.

How do you fight this anomaly during fasting? Try to distract yourself.

Try to pamper yourself. Personal care during fasting is my favorite strategy to kill time. Although fasting is difficult, take some time out to reward yourself. Immerse yourself in the tub with Epsom salts and read or listen to an interesting book. Go out and get a good haircut. Take a spa day. You're going through something incredibly difficult, and you deserve to be pampered.

Be organized. Organizing or cleaning around the house is another great distraction you could follow. For me, I always try to make lists of things during my non-fasting days that I'll do while fasting.

There are always little things we need to do around our home, office, and so on. They seem always to bother you but haven't made time for them. Now is your chance to take care of those bothersome errands. You could empty the messy closet that you've been using for years to be cleaned, clean and rearrange your storage cupboard, clean the dishes and wash your car, or delve into other chores. Some distractions that come with physical involvement can be very effective and also give you a light workout too.

Indulge Yourself. There's absolutely nothing embarrassing in engaging in unproductive activities to help you pass through a fast state because using few hours to play is better than giving up to achieve your desired result due to boredom. Watch videos on YouTube, watch your desired TV program, play games, and more.

I resort to checking my email, replying to Twitter or Facebook messages, whenever I feel bored and hungry. Normally, I would've stopped myself from doing these as it's unproductive, but I believe that it's better to be unproductive than to fail my fast because I know my health matters!

It's not difficult to realize when it's boredom that you're suffering from and not hunger. When you notice this, try to play around for some minutes to push through. Once the hunger vanishes, you can start your work again.

Go out for a walk. Most times, leaving the house or office is very helpful in keeping you going when you feel like giving up. You could decide to go to the store and buy some sparkling water, or tea, go and visit a friend. Even getting up to walk around the house or work with no aim in mind helps too.

When I reach the point that I'm doing this, I try to remember that my aim is my overall health and well-being. I imagine how happy I will be after achieving my goal and how people will feel after seeing me lose weight. Thinking of this while fresh air cools my frayed nerves keeps me inspired to move on with my fast.

Focus. By using your brain power effectively, your mind will automatically ignore thinking of food. Try to learn new things and put them into practice immediately like learning a new language or even a new hobby. Personally, I throw myself into a book or something that needs my full attention.

Nevertheless, the higher level of adrenaline and orexin in your system will help you to be up-and-doing, meaning your brain can take-in educative information easily and comfortably. Put it into practice, and you'll be surprised at how useful you can be with that extra time you're not worried over what to eat.

- Those times that you think you're hungry not knowing you're only bored

- Delve into your normal routine and get rid of boredom

Flee from Places Where You Can Smell or See Food

This reason made me break a lot of my fasts in the beginning. As I move on with my fasting confidently, thinking nothing will be able to stop me, I accidentally smell delicious food from somewhere. That very next moment I'd go for that meal and start eating, knowing I won't be happy with myself for the next 20 minutes. I suffered from this problem for quite a while, and I also know that it will happen again. I began to wonder the reason why I couldn't hold myself back since I knew it wasn't hunger, but I kept falling to that little test. So what was it?

We're are programmed in a way that if we see or smell food, we start salivating to it. Immediately our digestive system opens for food intake, and our mouths began to water. Before we know it, our brain starts screaming at us to Eat! Eat!! Eat now!!!

It will take you a monk's discipline to resist eating food. Even if you don't, don't beat yourself up too much about it. The easiest and only way to avoid this is to stay away from hot food in those few days of your fast. As those days pass, you would be in ketosis and resisting won't be challenging any longer.

If you're the type that cooks for other people like yourself, make them understand that you're in your fasting days and can't cook for those periods. If that isn't possible, you could buy takeout food or schedule preparing a meal for them during your non-fasting days.

- Being close to food will make your body want to eat

- Resisting the urge to eat is incredibly difficult when your brain is pushing you to eat something

Meditate

You can remove yourself from feelings of hunger by practicing meditation. Push yourself far away from the urge to eat until that cravings disappear.

One other best idea to eliminate hunger or craving for food is to shift your focus. Whether you're fasting or not, meditation helps greatly to rid your head-space, but together with fasting, meditation and fasting enhance and synergize each other.

- You're free to meditate at any point in time
- For beginners, it's healthy to practice guided meditation

Remember Why You Started

Always remember that you engaged in fasting for a purpose, and not for the sake that you don't feel like eating. Try to write the reasons that made you go into fasting, daily. What's that thing you want to change by fasting? Are you fasting for personal reasons? And why?

Try to write down the reasons you're fasting after doing it today. Do it tomorrow as well, because most people easily forget their reasons for doing something. Make it a habit of reminding yourself daily by writing it down as many times as possible so that it will be imprinted in your brain.

From now on anytime your memory tells you to eat it will immediately ring in your head that you're fasting.

- So write those reasons down so you'll know them by heart
- Don't forget that it's only you who can personally end the fast

Habit Changes

Anyone who fasts to lose weight and yet doesn't make any habit/diet changes will gradually recover all the weight used up during the fasting period

If your goal for doing a water fast is to lose weight, ensure your first focus is to change your eating habits, then gradually proceed to water fasting via the previously explained methods. Upon returning to your usual self, stick to your changed diet habit.

Old habits vs. New habits – begins with:

- Staying away from animal products: All dairy products, eggs, and meat. You'll shed so much weight by doing this, and it'll make you look and feel a lot better.

- Along with every meal, eat a big serving of green leafy salad.

- Include one freshly extracted vegetable juice in your everyday routine.

- Also, in your everyday meal plan, include activated charcoal and alkaline water in your diet.

- Engage in one short water fast every week, or intermittent water fast every month, or 3-day extended water fast every three months.

Following these steps will help you ensure success in stopping the old habits and keeping the new habits.

Chapter 10: Frequently Asked Questions

Who can fast?

For a few conditions, fasting is not recommended. During a fast, fatty acids are required as a substitute energy source, but a small percentage of people do not possess the enzyme that is necessary to metabolize fatty acids as a result of an inborn error of metabolism. A prolonged duration of fasting is not advisable for this set of people. An expert can quickly identify this inborn error at the start of fasting.

Certain conditions are not favorable to fasting, and they include; Pregnancy, some forms of cancer, use of some medications, kidney and liver disorders, severe weakness, and starvation.

How to know when to fast?

Knowing when to fast is dependent on your current health status and what you plan to achieve by fasting. For most people, taking up a complete change in diet, participating in a realistic exercise plan, getting adequate sleep, and living in a somewhat hygienic environment will contribute to the conditions necessary for restoration, and sustenance of vital health. Fasting can be very instrumental in promoting recovery especially when one is finding it hard to change their diet and lifestyle. Fasting can help to defeat addictions to recreational drugs like nicotine, alcohol, and caffeine, and stimulants like salt, sugar by re-adjusting the nervous system's sensitivity. Fasting has helped people appreciate the crude, natural taste of good food as you hear testimonials talking about romaine lettuce's sweetness, an apple's fresh taste, and the unbelievably rich taste of baked potatoes even without butter, and sour cream.

Some decide to fast without the apparent evidence of disease with the knowledge that a total physiological reset will cause the body to renew itself and rid itself of toxins accumulated in tissues despite our attempts at living right.

How long can you water fast for without causing any harm?

Depending on your experience with water fasting, I'd advise a first timer not to water fast for more than three days (72 hours).

It has been agreed in the community of water fasting that even though one might have some experience with fasting, water fasting for more than three days is best done under close supervision by medical experts in a fasting retreat.

This is unarguably true as there are several reasons why the retreat makes fasting much easier; those reasons are:

- The availability of a medical expert on call to answer all your questions

- There are no interruptions by any activities from your daily routine.

- The retreat is filled with people of like minds, also keen on fasting

The expensive fee for the fasting retreat, and sometimes the unwillingness of patients used to the idea of pausing one's daily routine for a couple of weeks is the sole drawback of a fasting retreat.

How frequently do I have to water fast?

To rejuvenate the immune system, one should embark on a 3-day fast quarterly (that is, every 12 weeks, or every three months) or it can be one only once a year for 7-10 days to lower the frequency of cancer incidences to a large extent.

What kind of water do I drink?

It is possible for one to have a disproportion of electrolytes and lack of minerals, in this case, it is advisable to drink mineral water. You should also drink sparkling water and regular water.

Is tea allowed during a water fast?

Pure water fasting involves water exclusively. It is not harmful if you add tea to your water fast and it might be helpful because it provides natural nutrients. Drink only tea containing water and avoid milk.

What amount of weight is lost on a water fast?

Each person is different, and only your body can determine how much you will lose. It is recommended that losing weight using water fasting should be done with the guidance of a doctor and weight loss should not exceed 1.1 kg (or two and a half pounds) every week.

Is it possible for me to lose muscle?

The majority of muscle loss occurs in the first 3-4 days of fasting, so it is generally dependent on the way you fast. Once your body begins to produce ketones as an alternative source of energy to glucose, the body is said to be in ketosis, and this attempt to save protein is what leads to the loss of muscle, albeit fairly small.

What is ketosis?

After eating the food eaten is turned into glucose which gives energy to the brain, muscles and other parts of the body. Your body makes use of the leftover glucose and starts to breakdown fatty acids in the liver to manufacture ketones when you've not eaten. During a fast, ketones are another form of energy which the body uses competently- the brain, heart, cells loves ketones, and they like ketones better (the primary source of energy of the heart are fatty acids). Ketosis is a state where ketones are the only source of energy used by the body.

What is the difference between juice fasting and water fasting?

Water fasting limits your intake to water exclusively, and sometimes tea; whereas a juice fast allows fruit juices and various vegetables. If correctly done, juice fasting increases your energy levels and maintain your blood glucose. Otherwise, it might result in fluctuations levels of blood sugar, and this can be dangerous.

Can I do a juice fast instead?

The purpose of water fasting is attaining and sustaining ketosis quickly, as ketosis helps you enjoy the benefits sooner. Even though juice fasting is beneficial too, the probability of reaching deep ketosis, or even reaching ketosis at all is low because of the higher sugar-water content compare to the fiber content.

Because of that difference, water fasting and juice fasting are not similar in any way.

How many glasses of water should I drink daily?

In a day, a range of 9-13 cups of water is ideal. ABOUT 13 glasses of water and fluids equivalent to 3 liters are ideal for men, and 9 cups equal to 2.2 liters is ideal for women. You can drink pure water available or water that has been distilled or simply continue with the recommended intake with regular tap water.

Try not to drink it all at a go! You could fill three 1-liter jugs to monitor the volume you are drinking and try to break your drinking into smaller quantities for the day.

Make sure not to drink more than the advised quantity of water daily because it can cause health problems since it creates an imbalance of minerals and salt in the body.

Fight hunger spells. Tackle hunger pains by consuming 1-2 cups of water then relax or take a nap if you're able; the urge to eat will generally pass. Also, meditation and reading a book can help take your mind off it.

Can I be productive during a fast?

For the initial five days in a 10-days fast, you will not think about doing much, so the best you can do is rest throughout that period. After the five days, you will be without strength, and there will be low blood pressure (postural hypertension- being unable to stand up fast), but you will possibly be motivated to read, work, learn or do other things because while in ketosis you'll feel psychologically energized. If you cannot schedule five or more days of rest, begin with a three-day water fast over a weekend or for five days beginning from Thursday and finishing on a Monday.

Won't I gain back more weight after a fast since my rate of metabolism will reduce while I'm fasting and after the fast?

Our time our physiological needs causes alterations in metabolic rate. During vigorous activities, our metabolic rate fires up and during rest/sleep our the metabolic rate declines. From this time, during a fast our metabolic rate declines because there's a reduction in physiological requirements compared to times when one is carrying out their routine activities and eating. Metabolic rate increases to correlate with rising physiological needs when a person breaks a fast and returns to their previous activities.

During a fast, the assimilative and digestive capacity is altered. A fast brings about the repair of the digestive organs hence optimizing nutrients intake. Gaining or losing weight is merely dependent on the number of calories taken in compared to the number broken down.

Can IBS be cured by water fasting?

Usually, the initial recommendation for IBS is frequent meals and diet patterns, and this is the best piece of advice that people with IBS are given. Although there is no long-term, direct research concerning fasting for people with IBS, there may be some issues for them.

First, fasting; particularly in the absence of professional guidance, might lead to a lowered intake of some nutrients in the diet, resulting in a high risk of nutritional imbalances.

Secondly, there is a reduction in the content of food such as fiber and probiotics that are specific to the gut, and this might reduce the number of bacteria that are beneficial to the gut.

Can kidney stones result from water fasting?

There are disparities in the studies carried out on the prevalence of kidney stones, renal colic, and urinary stones while on a fast. The outcomes of research in the connection between fasting and urinary stones are different and, in some cases, might be conflicting. Most research suggests that an increase in the incidence of urinary stones is not connected to fasting but is as a result of weather changes, increase in temperature and increased humidity. So, if you have a higher risk of developing a kidney stone, rather than engaging in extended fasting, I advise intermittent fasting as a better option.

Can ulcers result from water fasting?

There is no proof that fasting causes ulcers in the small intestine and stomach. Digestion of food is enhanced by the acids that are secreted by the stomach, and these acids are also protective against microorganisms. Mucus is also produced to protect the lining of the small intestine and stomach. Ulcers are caused by sores that result from the acid in the stomach acting on a reduced or worn out mucus lining that can no longer protect body tissues. This might occur in the intestine or stomach and is known as gastric ulcer or peptic ulcer.

Stomach ulcers result from long-term H.pylori infection and a reduction in the protective mucus lining of the stomach. There is a reduction in the mucous when

NSAIDs(nonsteroidal anti-inflammatory drugs) are used for a long time, since they inhibit inflammation, they also inhibit the production of mucus. It is doubtful that only fasting would result in ulcers, except in people with already existing gastritis and ulcers it could aggravate the symptoms.

A lot of people suffering from ulcers are relieved after drinking or eating while pain associated with an ulcer is made worse by many foods. Therefore, an ulcer is caused by bacteria, probably with NSAID use and highly unlikely with fasting. Consult your doctor. If you are on a drug to manage your ulcer, fasting is probably not for you.

Is an enema advisable?

Avoid getting an enema (colon cleansing) while in a water fast. Although there is a misconception that an enema is essential, science has discovered no proof that it is beneficial, it might even be harmful to your health. Enemas can result in, cramping, vomiting and bloating.

Conclusion

I used to practice one-day water fasting weekly during my twenties, and it was an enlightening experience that I remember well. Over time, those one-day fasts became easier to do, and I always felt refreshed and renewed.

As time moved along and the older I got, I had stumbled across other ways to rid myself of toxins besides water fasting; such as the intake of cleansing herbs for my colon and complete body cleansing, routine raw vegan meals, occasional fasting from meals.

The processes such as repairing and detoxifying that happens while fasting also happens when a person is actively consuming meals. For people whose conditions are not getting better as quickly as they want it to or those that need a specific time of healing for resolution, a fast can be greatly beneficial. It is also important to note that it is a person's lifestyle after the fast that is the most crucial aspect of the fast. Fasting gives a fresh and renewed baseline to develop a flourishing body by regularly choosing to eat healthily and live right.

For detoxification, and other health benefits I still personally rely on short term and periodic water fasting over the course of a meal, a day, or even a few days.

Water fasting for more than three days needs detailed planning (before and after), self-education and also professional assistance as required.

Fasting can be an arduous ordeal, depending on one's health, emotional and mental state.

Hence, I recommend that before, during, and after a fast consider the physical advantages of the fast over your overall state of health. Knowing this will reduce the acute stress produced by those adverse effects which obviously does not boost your health and make you feel better.

Water fasting is one of the most natural diets on earth if you follow the most crucial rule of consuming adequate water throughout the fast and some other additional tips like not standing up too fast.

Remember that that water fasting may be simple does not make it easy.

Other diets do not genuinely remove hunger, and this is the significant advantage that water fasting has over diets – if you water fast properly hunger is completely eliminated.

Reference

1. Zimmer, C. (2019). Self-Destructive Behavior in Cells May Hold Key to a Longer Life. Retrieved from https://www.nytimes.com/2009/10/06/science/06cell.html?pagewanted=all&_r=1

2. Ohsumi, Y. (2013). Historical landmarks of autophagy research. Cell Research, 24(1), 9-23. doi: 10.1038/cr.2013.169

3. Autophagy 101: How Intermittent Fasting Could Help Us Age Slowly. (2019). Retrieved from https://thechalkboardmag.com/what-is-autophagy-intermittent-fasting-process

4. Madeo, F., Zimmermann, A., Maiuri, M., & Kroemer, G. (2015). Essential role for autophagy in life span extension. Journal Of Clinical Investigation, 125(1), 85-93. doi: 10.1172/jci73946

5. Shetty, A., Kodali, M., Upadhya, R., & Madhu, L. (2018). Emerging Anti-Aging Strategies - Scientific Basis and Efficacy. Aging And Disease, 9(6), 1165. doi: 10.14336/ad.2018.1026

6. Mizushima, N., Yoshimori, T., & Ohsumi, Y. (2011). The Role of Atg Proteins in Autophagosome Formation. Annual Review Of Cell And Developmental Biology, 27(1), 107-132. doi: 10.1146/annurev-cellbio-092910-154005

7. Mizushima, N., Ohsumi, Y., & Yoshimori, T. (2002). Autophagosome Formation in Mammalian Cells. Cell Structure And Function, 27(6), 421-429. doi: 10.1247/csf.27.421

8. Castro-Obregon, S. (2019). Lysosomes, Autophagy | Learn Science at Scitable. Retrieved from https://www.nature.com/scitable/topicpage/the-discovery-of-lysosomes-and-autophagy-14199828

9. Bandyopadhyay, U., Kaushik, S., Varticovski, L., & Cuervo, A. (2008). The Chaperone-Mediated Autophagy Receptor Organizes in Dynamic Protein Complexes at the Lysosomal Membrane. Molecular And Cellular Biology, 28(18), 5747-5763. doi: 10.1128/mcb.02070-07

10. Gump, J., & Thorburn, A. (2011). Autophagy and apoptosis: what is the connection?. Trends In Cell Biology, 21(7), 387-392. doi: 10.1016/j.tcb.2011.03.007

11. Alirezaei, M., Kemball, C., Flynn, C., Wood, M., Whitton, J., & Kiosses, W. (2010). Short-term fasting induces profound neuronal autophagy. Autophagy, 6(6), 702-710. doi: 10.4161/auto.6.6.12376

12. He, C., Sumpter, Jr., R., & Levine, B. (2012). Exercise induces autophagy in peripheral tissues and in the brain. Autophagy, 8(10), 1548-1551. doi: 10.4161/auto.21327

13. Land, S. (2019). Mistruths and Lies About Autophagy. Retrieved from https://siimland.com/mistruths-and-lies-about-autophagy/

14. Westerterp, K. (2004). Nutrition & Metabolism, 1(1), 5. doi: 10.1186/1743-7075-1-5

15. Bellisle F, e. (2019). Meal frequency and energy balance. - PubMed - NCBI. Retrieved from https://www.ncbi.nlm.nih.gov/pubmed/9155494

16. Smeets, A., & Westerterp-Plantenga, M. (2007). Acute effects on metabolism and appetite profile of one meal difference in the lower range of meal frequency. British Journal Of Nutrition, 99(06). doi: 10.1017/s0007114507877646

17. Leidy, H., Armstrong, C., Tang, M., Mattes, R., & Campbell, W. (2010). The Influence of Higher Protein Intake and Greater Eating Frequency on Appetite Control in Overweight and Obese Men. Obesity, 18(9), 1725-1732. doi: 10.1038/oby.2010.45

18. SPEECHLY, D., & BUFFENSTEIN, R. (1999). Greater Appetite Control Associated with an Increased Frequency of Eating in Lean Males. Appetite, 33(3), 285-297. doi: 10.1006/appe.1999.0265

19. Jon Schoenfeld, B., Albert Aragon, A., & Krieger, J. (2015). Effects of meal frequency on weight loss and body composition: a meta-analysis. Nutrition Reviews, 73(2), 69-82. doi: 10.1093/nutrit/nuu017

20. Cameron, J., Cyr, M., & Doucet, É. (2009). Increased meal frequency does not promote greater weight loss in subjects who were prescribed an 8-week equi-energetic energy-restricted diet. British Journal Of Nutrition, 1. doi: 10.1017/s0007114509992984

21. Alirezaei, M., Kemball, C., Flynn, C., Wood, M., Whitton, J., & Kiosses, W. (2010). Short-term fasting induces profound neuronal autophagy. Autophagy, 6(6), 702-710. doi: 10.4161/auto.6.6.12376

22. Koopman, K., Caan, M., Nederveen, A., Pels, A., Ackermans, M., & Fliers, E. et al. (2014). Hypercaloric diets with increased meal frequency, but not meal size,

increase intrahepatic triglycerides: A randomized controlled trial. Hepatology, 60(2), 545-553. doi: 10.1002/hep.27149

23. de Verdier, M., & Longnecker, M. (1992). Eating frequency—a neglected risk factor for colon cancer?. Cancer Causes & Control, 3(1), 77-81. doi: 10.1007/bf00051916

24. Heilbronn, L., Smith, S., Martin, C., Anton, S., & Ravussin, E. (2005). Alternate-day fasting in nonobese subjects: effects on body weight, body composition, and energy metabolism. The American Journal Of Clinical Nutrition, 81(1), 69-73. doi: 10.1093/ajcn/81.1.69

25. Arnal, M., Mosoni, L., Boirie, Y., Houlier, M., Morin, L., & Verdier, E. et al. (1999). Protein pulse feeding improves protein retention in elderly women. The American Journal Of Clinical Nutrition, 69(6), 1202-1208. doi: 10.1093/ajcn/69.6.1202

26. Varady, K. (2011). Intermittent versus daily calorie restriction: which diet regimen is more effective for weight loss?. Obesity Reviews, 12(7), e593-e601. doi: 10.1111/j.1467-789x.2011.00873.x

27. Stote, K., Baer, D., Spears, K., Paul, D., Harris, G., & Rumpler, W. et al. (2007). A controlled trial of reduced meal frequency without caloric restriction in healthy, normal-weight, middle-aged adults. The American Journal Of Clinical Nutrition, 85(4), 981-988. doi: 10.1093/ajcn/85.4.981

28. Barnosky, A., Hoddy, K., Unterman, T., & Varady, K. (2014). Intermittent fasting vs daily calorie restriction for type 2 diabetes prevention: a review of human findings. Translational Research, 164(4), 302-311. doi: 10.1016/j.trsl.2014.05.013

29. 5 Day Water Fast: What to Expect on the Healing Journey - DrJockers.com. (2019). Retrieved from https://drjockers.com/water-fast/

30. Water Fasting: 12 Strategies to Prepare Properly - DrJockers.com. (2019). Retrieved from https://drjockers.com/water-fasting/

31. Cheng, C., Adams, G., Perin, L., Wei, M., Zhou, X., & Lam, B. et al. (2014). Prolonged Fasting Reduces IGF-1/PKA to Promote Hematopoietic-Stem-Cell-Based Regeneration and Reverse Immunosuppression. Cell Stem Cell, 14(6), 810-823. doi: 10.1016/j.stem.2014.04.014

32. Paoli, A. (2014). Ketogenic Diet for Obesity: Friend or Foe?. International Journal Of Environmental Research And Public Health, 11(2), 2092-2107. doi: 10.3390/ijerph110202092

33. Takagi, A., Kume, S., Maegawa, H., & Uzu, T. (2016). Emerging role of mammalian autophagy in ketogenesis to overcome starvation. Autophagy, 12(4), 709-710. doi: 10.1080/15548627.2016.1151597

34. Varady, K., Bhutani, S., Church, E., & Klempel, M. (2009). Short-term modified alternate-day fasting: a novel dietary strategy for weight loss and cardioprotection in obese adults. The American Journal Of Clinical Nutrition, 90(5), 1138-1143. doi: 10.3945/ajcn.2009.28380

35. Heilbronn, L., Smith, S., Martin, C., Anton, S., & Ravussin, E. (2005). Alternate-day fasting in nonobese subjects: effects on body weight, body composition, and energy metabolism. The American Journal Of Clinical Nutrition, 81(1), 69-73. doi: 10.1093/ajcn/81.1.69

36. Cava, E., Yeat, N., & Mittendorfer, B. (2017). Preserving Healthy Muscle during Weight Loss. Advances In Nutrition: An International Review Journal, 8(3), 511-519. doi: 10.3945/an.116.014506

37. Leidy, H., Mattes, R., & Campbell, W. (2007). Effects of Acute and Chronic Protein Intake on Metabolism, Appetite, and Ghrelin During Weight Loss*. Obesity, 15(5), 1215-1225. doi: 10.1038/oby.2007.143